Life to the Years

LIFE TO THE
YEARS

Living a Robust Life
After Heart Disease

MICHAEL JAMES DO, FACC,
& MICHAEL RANVILLE

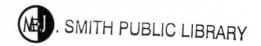 . SMITH PUBLIC LIBRARY

NEW YORK

LONDON • NASHVILLE • MELBOURNE • VANCOUVER

LIFE TO THE YEARS:

Living a Robust Life After Heart Disease

Published in New York, New York, by Morgan James Publishing. Morgan James is a trademark of Morgan James, LLC. www.MorganJamesPublishing.com

The Morgan James Speakers Group can bring authors to your live event. For more information or to book an event visit The Morgan James Speakers Group at www.TheMorganJamesSpeakersGroup.com.

ISBN 9781683507710 paperback
ISBN 9781683507727 eBook
Library of Congress Control Number: 2017914683

Cover Design by:
Megan Whitney
megan@creativeninjadesigns.com

Interior Design by:
Chris Treccani
www.3dogcreative.net

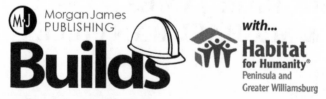

In an effort to support local communities, raise awareness and funds, Morgan James Publishing donates a percentage of all book sales for the life of each book to Habitat for Humanity Peninsula and Greater Williamsburg.

Get involved today! Visit
www.MorganJamesBuilds.com

DEDICATION

Michael J. James, DO, FACC:

To all my patients; past, present and future: I am the true beneficiary of the life added to your years.

To all my students, Residents and Fellows that may have picked up a Pearl or two that added life to your patients' years.

Michael W. Ranville:

To Carol and Mara: I will forever cherish the memory of waking from the long sleep of surgery to the sight of your strong and reassuring smiles.

OTHER WORKS

Also by Michael James, DO, FACC

Dr. Michael James is a Senior Partner at the Thoracic Cardiovascular Institute. He has served as a Clinical Professor on the faculty at Michigan State University since 1982.

Lavin, L. Gonzales, Chi, S, Baird, W, James, M.J., Sparrow, A, "How Michigan State University's Cooperative Heart Program Enhances University Community Education"—Michigan Medicine, September 1977

James, M.J, Das, S.U., "Cardiomyopathy—A Plea for Optimism", Practical Cardiology, October 1976

James, M.J, "Clinical Spectrum of Sinus Node Disease Sick Sinus Syndrome," JAOA, 73: April 1974

James, M.J., Haspel, L.U., "Experience with Coronary Care Unit Analysis of 120 Cases", the DO, July 1973

James, M.J., "Parental Hyperalimentation" JAOA, 71: February 1972

James, M.J, Brandt, R., "Infected Left Atrial Myxoma: Report of a Case"

Also by Michael Ranville

Michael Ranville is the author of numerous magazine articles on such diverse topics as politics, sports and humor.

"To Strike at a King: the Turning Point in the McCarthy Witch-Hunts"

PREFACE

"The mass of men lead lives of quiet desperation..."
HENRY DAVID THOREAU—WALDEN

Michael James, DO:

I am a cardiologist. Taking care of heart patients is I all I ever wanted to do. My career has known both success and desperation. The success is easily traced to the patients I have returned to a normal and productive life, like my writing partner, Michael Ranville. Mike's tenacity, coupled with a refusal to accept a sedentary life style, speaks to the hope heart patients now have for a productive life. The desperation is borne of knowing that ultimately medicine is finite. No patient is routine.

Viewing my near fifty years in medicine I can state without equivocation, desperation finishes a distant second to sense of accomplishment.

There is more to the famous Thoreau quote; lesser known but equally significant. In its entirety it reads, "The mass of men lead lives of quiet desperation, *and go to the grave with the song still in them.*" The pages ahead represent the song I chose not to take to my grave.

In 1905, heart disease replaced tuberculosis and pneumonia as the leading killer in the United States. More than a century later it has yet to relinquish that dubious distinction. My career in cardiology, and this book, is driven by that unyielding statistic. Writing from different perspectives, Mike and I believe there is merit in a letter of accomplishment from the cardiac community that heart disease, however lethal its history, no longer translates into a tranquil life bereft of passion and achievement.

Our message is fashioned first and foremost for heart patients and their families. Thanks to an explosion of research and technology over the past fifty years, heart patients are no longer consigned to live out their days in an easy chair, robbed of dignity, lethargically watching daytime television while a resentful family is conscripted into the role of caretaker. That message is accompanied by the compelling stories of those whose insight and foresight drove that research and technology.

We also train our message on the cardiac care community. The mission has changed dramatically over the past fifty years. Where once our goal was to make heart patients comfortable, we now are charged with preparing them for re-entry into the workforce, and assuming full workloads and responsibilities once they have arrived. It is an honorable and rewarding mission, and it is succeeding.

The idea of a dual perspective approach was conceived with my writing partner, patient, and friend Mike Ranville. I kept abreast of the meteoric advances in cardiac research and technology through the years; upon presentation to Mike, he willingly embraced them. He quickly and convincingly eschewed the easy chair and daytime television in favor of a return to work and a robust career in a high pressure environment. Heart patients, and the families of heart patients, will find his comments motivating, useful and interesting.

Medical students may also take comfort in my struggle with standardized tests. By all accounts my career has been a success. Yet an inability to master the elusive task of doing well on a standardized test was responsible for a number of obstacles that were overcome only by dogged determination.

As we were writing the book, Mike underwent a heart transplant and encountered a confrontation with his own mortality. The transplant prompted our candid examination of end-of-life decisions from the perspectives of doctor, patient and family.

The book is far more than the story of a doctor-patient relationship. It explores the history of cardiac care, and how the heart attacks incurred by two U.S. Presidents—Warren Harding and Dwight D. Eisenhower – shaped public opinion of heart disease for many years. The efforts to conceal the severity of their heart problems from the public proved pivotal to the federal government's lack of involvement in combating the nation's number one killer.

We cite the indefatigable efforts of Mary Lasker and her legendary fact sheet that provided the catalyst for the federal government's decision to finally become involved in the war against the nation's number one killer. A fascinating person unto herself, Mary Lasker, and her impressive array of personal contacts, marshalled the effort for federal involvement.

We also enlisted the talented pens of Pam Nyquist and my colleague Dr. David Strobl, DO. Pam tells the compelling story of her father, and my patient and good friend, the memorable Ed Hardin, former President of Michigan State University. Ed Hardin's final days form the backdrop of our chapter on the pivotal role dignity plays in end-of-life decisions.

Dr. David Strobl, DO, offers his unique insights into diet, the critical component of heart care. His approach to healthy eating, pared of complex weighing of items in columns A and B, will please many and offer comfort to those who continually equivocate—"I just don't have the will power for a diet." Dr. Strobl calmly offers, "Just meet me halfway."

Michael Ranville:

I accepted Dr. James challenge to join him and co-author a book on heart disease—or more accurately, living with heart disease—because he convinced me that my story could inspire other heart patients to rise from the easy chair and embrace an active life. If telling my story achieves that goal for just one patient then the effort will have been a success.

I had no idea my conversations with Dr. James would lead to a book. Evidently, far too often we went beyond the time allotted for my office visit. Such was my growing reputation for tying up the boss's schedule, upon arrival for appointments, his staff would gently remind me, "Dr. James is running tight today."

At first we talked about writing an article together, usually involving his less than gracious regard for colleagues who rarely look up from their computers during appointments. "There's an actual person sitting in front of you," he would rant, "a person whose appointment with you has been circled on the refrigerator calendar for the past month, a person whose family and friends want to know, 'What did the doctor say?' We owe them more than the top of our heads."

I loved his passion for medicine and his patients.

I was forty years old when I had a heart attack. I fully appreciated his blunt, unvarnished approach to my cardiac care program. He let me know, "It's okay to sweat again." And sweat I did. I resumed all physical activity—the softball team with my buddies, the water skiing with my daughter, even took up running…well okay, jogging. I went back to work at a pressure-laden job; thankfully, no coddling there.

In addition to a full schedule at work, I also began pursuit of a life-long dream to write. I had always written for the job – speeches, reports, etc.—but now I was writing for myself; my topic of choice—and most importantly, my byline. Long days that frequently stretched into long nights were the norm. But I was producing, not taking. And I was not holding forth from that wretched easy chair.

I thrived under Dr. James care. He loved the fact that I was leading a vigorous life; it buttressed his belief that heart patients are capable of leading strong, independent lives. He was totally supportive of my pushing the envelope regarding physical activity and stress. I was feeling better than I had in years.

My activity level prompted discussion of letting others know there was life after a heart attack. The ability to engage life at its fullest was the product of Dr. James's willingness to keep current with the research and my willingness to embrace Coach James's game plan.

After a year or so of talking about it, we both concluded, "Talk's cheap." We began to write, wandering about at first, but soon structure appeared.

Writers are not known for "working and playing well with others," but between his appointments and my now-active schedule we hit a stride.

We harbor no illusions of challenging James Patterson's stranglehold on the New York Times Bestsellers. But we are enthused at the prospect of our effort being instrumental in motivating heart patients to add life to their remaining years.

TABLE OF CONTENTS

FOREWORD

Dr. Clarence Lasby

Life to the Years is a masterful and compelling account of the relationship of a doctor and his patient in combating and adjusting to heart disease, the number one killer of Americans for more than a century. The authors' mission is to convince their readers that the long-held view of a heart disease as a harbinger of death or life as a cardiac cripple is no longer relevant, and that fifty years of exceptional progress in cardiology offer the promise, indeed the likelihood, of a vigorous and productive life. Their gripping personal story of working together to confront an array of cardiac events, from heart attack to atrial fibrillation to implants and finally a heart transplant, and with lasting success, confirms their message of hope. It also provides a framework for inquiries into a host of related issues—historical events including the misdiagnosis of two presidents, current research on cardiac drugs, procedures and diet, and the complexity of end of life discussions—always addressed with insight, honesty and humanity. As a student of the history of medicine and a cardiac patient for more than four decades, I found this book enlightening and uplifting, a gift to any reader.

CHAPTER ONE:

"Requiescat in Pace— Let Dignity Prevail"

"As physicians it is our job to add life to years, not years to life."
—UNKNOWN, FIRST HEARD BY DR. JAMES IN A CLASS
TAUGHT BY DR. LEO STEIN

Dr. Michael James:

Life is full of stark realities, chief among them people don't live forever. If a physician prefers to avoid the angst that accompanies dealing with terminal patients, then better a career teaching love sonnets of the Elizabethan era. Miracles happen—mostly in the Bible, though, rarely in a hospital room. Despite the most fervent wishes and desperate prayers of an anxious family, modern medicine, no matter how sophisticated or advanced, does not confer immortality.

The vast majority of the pages ahead deal with reducing misery and preserving life. However, underscoring that premise is the persistent notion that quality is the essential ingredient of that preserved life, not just time. I vividly recall the profound observation of Dr. Leo Stein, my pathology professor at the Chicago College of Osteopathic Medicine, "As physicians," he observed, "it is our job to add life to the years, not years to the life."

Dr. Stein was blunt; we never had to wrestle with deciphering his intent. While some were put off, even offended, with his brusque nature, I admired it. His point still resonates forty-five years after class adjourned that day, and that speaks volumes to the telling impact his message wielded. My professional demeanor today reflects the admiration and respect I hold for Dr. Stein, in particular his ability to chart a quick and accurate path to the heart of a diagnosis.

End of life situations involve straddling a frequently elusive line between sorely needed candor and the natural desire to offer comfort. Unfortunately, medical schools shy from discussing physician deportment regarding end of life decisions. Dr. Stein's lecture was the closest I received in my medical training. That was 1970. And now, nearly fifty years later, despite the fact that the majority of health care dollars are spent on patients who are in the last two years of life, some physicians still take the circuitous route and only participate from the periphery in the "life to the years" versus the "years to the life" discussion.

But not all.

I didn't realize it at the time but Dr. Stein's message would have a similar impact on the next generation of physicians, and save me money in the process. Not long ago, after attending a delightful production at the Wharton Center for Performing Arts on the campus of Michigan State University, I was backing out of my parking space. Thinking I was clear, I felt the sickening crunch of my car butting into another. Jumping out, I quickly discerned this wasn't just any car I hit, it was a Porsche. Feeling stupid and embarrassed, I profoundly apologized, and wrote down my name and phone number. Examining the damaged rear fender of the otherwise immaculate Porsche, I was sure the repair figure would easily be in the five-figure range.

The Porsche owner looked at me and asked if I was the Dr. James who taught Cardiology at MSU.

"Yes I am."

"You lectured me at med school. I will always remember you stressing the importance of adding life to a patient's years, not just years to the life."

"I'm flattered you remember," I said, "but I need to pay for my stupidity here." He flatly rejected any attempt on my part to assume responsibility for the damaged fender.

"No way," he protested, "your lectures, especially the one dealing with 'life to years', governed my medical career. I'll take care of the car. You've given me so much more. Thank you."

Obviously, I was grateful the family exchequer would not suffer the consequences of my momentary loss of concentration in a parking lot. However, I was humbled and gratified to learn that an essential point of my medical instruction had been passed on, totally intact, to the next generation.

End of life is a trying time for all, especially to those members of the family charged with deciding if or when the ventilator is removed. The tools of medicine are finite. If the physician is less than candid regarding the assignment of resources that do nothing but enable the lingering to continue, and do nothing but add years to the life, then families are deprived of critical information essential to a critical decision.

It is a time when irrevocable decisions are frequently revoked. Many families or patients change their mind, one way or another, when the actual moment arrives to decide life or death. The fact that many patients deteriorate physically but maintain firm control of their mental faculties renders the decision even more difficult. Some harbor unrealistic expectations of recovery. They are in the hospital, and hospitals are where people heal. Coupled with a fear of the unknown, they conclude additional time will translate into recovery. Others want all artificial means of sustaining life removed, their decision driven by preserving personal dignity and ridding themselves of pain and discomfort.

If the decision is made to continue life support, it has to be accompanied by a reasonable expectation that some form of recovery is in the offing. In addition, if a recovery can reasonably be assumed, the quality of life that awaits the patient becomes paramount. Given that the patient is already infirmed, will the resumed life be different? Will it involve a dreaded increase in dependence on others? For some, the natural fear of death is outweighed by surrendering the loss of control and the quality of life that would be realized.

Other factors also influence the decision. Nursing homes and extended care facilities are of necessity governed by a rigid daily regimen. Many patients admittedly find comfort in a predictable schedule. Others, however, chafe at the inflexible framework. The loss of independence becomes far more than theory; it is real. You don't eat what you want or when you want, or even when you're hungry, but when the dinner bell rings. And it rings without fail at the same time every day. The spontaneity that may have been a cherished cornerstone of life is now subordinated to the need for conformity. Conveniences that were once an assumed part of daily life – brewing a cup of tea for instance—now fall under a by permission only directive. Frequently a roommate is assigned, adding a loss of valued privacy and even more discomfort to a life already disrupted. Autonomy becomes a less attainable goal with each passing day.

Moreover, there is a social stigma attached to the home, made worse by comedians sorely lacking in creativity mining for laughs with shallow, dementia-oriented humor. While Jonathan Winters just might be one of the funniest comedians ever, his admittedly popular dementia-laden character, "Maude Frickert", may pass as humor to some, but to others is tasteless and cruel. Humor that plays on the loss of dignity brought on by age is not funny.

Taking up residence in the nursing home also quickly translates as the final stop before death. Family knows it, and in most cases, the patient does as well. In the not too distant past, the patient was fulfilling an obligation to visit family or friends residing in a nursing home. Now the patient has become the obligation.

Little wonder that some patients refuse to prolong life artificially; the loss of dignity that accompanies the alternative is not tenable. The family remembers a vibrant dad always ready for a few turns around the lake on water skis, or a game of catch in the backyard before supper. If you had a problem, Mom's gentle strength was always there; her bottomless pit of homespun wisdom at the ready to offer a great solution. However, there comes a time when Dad's days of playing catch are a thing of the past, when Mom is no longer capable and must look to others for the wisdom she once dispensed. No one wants to bear the responsibility of acknowledging the obvious; that the incessant pumping of the respirator is only adding years—or more accurately days or hours—to what was once a productive life.

Instead, the indecisive family turns to the physician. "Tell us what to do, doctor." And all this after a careful explanation pointing out that Dad is not going to get better. Sadly, there are few, if any, profiles in courage in a hospital room with a terminal patient.

The problem is compounded by those who fully expect, who demand, a miracle. In that same hospital room, reality can be elusive. "Doctor, that's my momma. You better do everything you can to make sure she lives."

The family dynamics of the final hours can run the gamut of emotions. While all claim to want what is best for the patient, love and fond memories color thoughtful decision-making. Should the loved one suffer? Should valuable and expensive resources be expended to prolong the inevitable? Is the person being kept alive by the respirator the same person who once played catch before supper or solved family problems, big and small, with insightful, homespun wisdom?

Avoidance of the decision frequently stems from guilt for things said and done that cannot be retracted at this late date. Weighing just as heavy is the concern for things not said and done – opportunities that will never be available again. And make no mistake; callous though it may be, death frequently brings out the avarice in a family. Some of what was not said and done is rooted in a fear that too little too late will be reflected in the will. Death strains a family in many ways.

Not to trivialize dying, but it would be so much easier if only we could chart life on a graph. At birth we would be awarded so many heartbeats. Perhaps a heartbeat meter could be fashioned to inform us at any point in time how many beats of the heart remain. Do we have enough time left to take that trip to Europe, to write that novel? Consult the heartbeat meter. Later in the book, we discuss the important role genes play in determining cardiac health. We sound the need to be more judicious in selecting parents. Key to the number of heartbeats initially assigned would be family history.

Lifestyle could be factored into increasing or decreasing the number of heartbeats. For instance, a carefully constructed diet, strictly adhered to, would add heartbeats; conversely, pizzas and Big Macs would reduce them. A calorie counter could be created; the fewer calories ingested the less chance for obesity and diabetes, hence more heartbeats. Regular exercise would be rewarded. The better the physical condition, the fewer heartbeats would be expended, thereby reducing the frequency of withdrawals from the heartbeat bank. While the heartbeat meter still awaits discovery, the factors that control the number of heartbeats are very real. But even those who have led the healthiest of lives, the number of heartbeats eventually draws down to a precious few. Knowing the problem is one thing.

Maybe we can at least begin quantifying the factors surrounding death. We learn more every day. There are some aspects regarding end-of-life that contain a degree of predictability. For instance, one emerging pattern beginning to draw attention is that end of life patients incur approximately seven crises before they die; some more, some less, but the average approaching seven. With each crisis the downhill slide grows steeper, affecting the "life to years" factor. Regardless, the original pre-crises state of health is never again realized.

More often than not, the final days are accompanied by discomfort; it is the nature of dying. Unfortunately, the discomfort is visited on those least able to tolerate it. Cancer patients are in pain; heart patients can't breathe. Neither is conducive to a peaceful passing. Melding the number of crises with the discomfort inherent in dying, might someday result in being able to quantify the factors involved in the decision to turn off the respirator.

Time takes its toll. The "heartbeat meter", like the life it chronicles, one day flashes the inevitable time for decision notice. Are the final heartbeats going to be recorded wearing a hospital gown watching daytime television? Or will they occur in the company of those who have enriched the life in question and provided cherished memories? Children, grandchildren, a show in Vegas—the options are as countless as the variety that characterized that life.

My writing partner, Mike Ranville, recounts a poignant moment. One of his clients was the Detroit Tigers. As might be expected, he was frequently put upon for tickets. One such request, though, stood out: a young woman he knew from working in the state capitol contacted him. She asked for fifteen tickets and insisted on paying for them, an unusual stipulation when providing tickets for those in the political arena. Her father, she explained, was in the final stages of cancer, his time measured in weeks, maybe even days.

She explained that her dad loved baseball, especially the Detroit Tigers. Despite the numbing medication, he could still follow the endless machinations in the drama that resides with every pitch in a major league baseball game. The ballgame would likely be his last. Family was his other love. Nothing made him happier than to be surrounded by his children and grandchildren. The fifteen tickets would allow him one final grand and glorious day with the people he loved, enjoying the game he loved. The Tigers were able to accommodate such a worthy request and helped secure fifteen seats in the same section, not an easy task.

Two weeks later Mike received a letter from the young woman thanking him for the tickets. Her father had died a few days after the game. The letter included a photo taken at the stadium. At the center of the picture was Dad, adorned in a cap emblazoned with the iconic Detroit Tigers Olde English D, surrounded by family, hoisting a beer and sporting a wide grin. Far from sad, her letter indicated during the days just before and after the funeral, the family repeatedly returned to that last game and the great memory they all had of the day. She pointed out it was the last time her dad really felt good. The picture was signed by all in attendance, including the guest of honor himself.

Did the outing shorten his life; zap him of strength that would have given him another day or so languishing in bed? Who knows? He chose one more enduring memory, a moment his family could always cherish; a memory that included a cold beer and the beautiful sounds of the ballpark; the crack of the bat, the roar of the crowd. The Tigers even cooperated by delivering a win.

There are those, both family and friends, who have confided in me their abhorrence at the thought of slowly deteriorating in a hospital bed, a nursing home, or in an Alzheimer's unit, bereft of dignity. If only the inevitable could be accomplished through sudden death, certainly my choice. But that's not always an option. What should be strived for, though, is the opportunity to ring your curtain down with class, to gather family and friends about you to fashion one final memory. Be it a day at the ballpark, a trip to the beach, or just sharing stories over a bottle of wine, it would be a moment of your choosing.

Atul Gawande, surgeon and writer, eloquently recorded his observations surrounding the end of life. His book, *Being Mortal*, is currently being devoured by the medical community. It is a riveting and perceptive recitation of the factors surrounding death. It should be required reading for physicians. Much of what he presents is familiar, or at the very least obvious. Physicians are healers, trained to fix things. What happens, though, when fixing things is no longer possible? While not the ideal, many of the decisions become individualized and rooted in the personal beliefs of the physician, and are profoundly affected by the degree that physician is willing to embrace candor. Protocols thrive in the medical community. Evidence Based Medicine abounds. Electronic Medical Records have prompts alerting the provider to tell a smoker not to smoke, to tell obese people to lose weight. No insightful brilliance there.

But what happens when those protocols confront the imprecise, when the things in our medical tool-kit we've relied on for years no longer help? The shrinking role of the family physician, (dealt with later in this book), is responsible for punting the decision on what to do next to the next man up – the hospitalist, the intensivist, the oncologist, the surgeon, the cardiologist—none of whom may have sufficient knowledge to know how the patient or family feels regarding the degree to which life should be prolonged. Our system is not equipped to address that crucial question. Sadly, no matter how futile the expected outcome, there is a sentiment of why not try one more procedure, one more test? Insurance is paying for it anyway.

Further, medical practices are increasingly being purchased by hospitals. If a patient's condition falls into the need for a discussion, and it's on a Friday, why not let the person in charge of rounds on Monday make the call. The sad but true tenet that hovers over many political deliberations—"They can't hang you for the decision you never make"—is alive and well in the medical community.

Mike Ranville and I are both products of a Catholic upbringing, raised in the carefully ingrained notion that "Life is a gift from God to be preserved at all costs." The Catholic Church used to administer the sacrament of Extreme Unction, the so-called "last rites," a special blessing for those deemed to be near death. While it had the benefit of serving notice that the time had come for the patient to put both the spiritual as well as the temporal house in order, it also helped ease acceptance of the inevitable. There was comfort in knowing you were at peace with your God.

I Know From Whence I Speak

My comments and observations are based on far more than just theory. I have watched both my parents and my wife's mother go through a lingering end of life. Being a physician, and, in their eyes, possessed with the ability to heal, made it even more frustrating.

My wife's mother accepted the fact that her days were numbered. My admiration for her is immense. While in a weakened state, she still controlled her final request – a hot dog and a Margarita.

The deaths of my parents were stressful. My father, Bernie James, was a *man's man* who moved about in life with a certain swagger and cast a long, dominating shadow right up to the end.

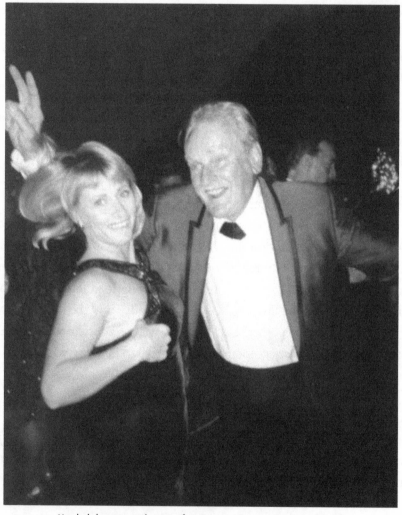

My dad dancing with my wife. Bernie James was a *man's man* who moved about in life with a certain swagger."

He slowly developed dementia, and would get lost coming home from the golf course or the corner tavern. On occasion, he arrived home escorted by his old firefighter buddies or local police officers who remembered Bernie when he was still bringing his A-game. It became painfully evident that my mother was not able to care for him.

There was a time in the not too distant past when he would just move in with one of his kids; in this case, my home was the logical choice. Like generations before us, we would take care of him, no questions asked. That was the natural progression of things. Growing up, many of my friends had grandparents living with them. But times change. We certainly had enough room and the financial means to ensure his comfort. But attending to his needs was a full-time job, the lion's share of which would fall to my wife while I was working. Given the dementia, his care would be even more demanding. Besides, where would my mother live?

We placed him in an Alzheimer's unit where he did little more than exist for two years. Visiting him was a gut-wrenching experience. Here was a firefighter, hailed as a hero throughout Cleveland for saving the life of an infant. Here was a man who was a commanding presence in my life, and the lives of many others as well. Here was a man of noteworthy accomplishments all borne of calloused hands and an indomitable spirit. Now here was that same man, diapered, fed and rolled around in a stroller. I was consumed with anger, disgust, and guilt. Bernie James's dignity was not a flexible feast, and neither would mine be, I vowed, when the time came. A deteriorating life is wretched to watch. Reality prevailed: Mom was relieved when dad died. Sadly, my Dad's sister made Mom feel guilty about putting her husband in an Alzheimer's unit. We reassured Mom there simply was no other choice.

My sister Bonnie had a strong relationship with my mother and after church spent most Sundays with her; taking her shopping, getting her nails done, her hair permed and other things designed to make her feel good about herself. When you look good, you feel good—and mom was looking good. Toward the end, the two of them traveled extensively. Disneyland was a favorite, as was Las Vegas—a great way to tell the world to go to hell and spend down to the last penny.

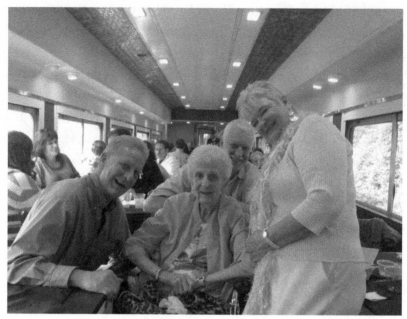

James family gathered around Mom. From left: Mark, Mom, Me, Bonnie.
"When you look good you feel good, and mom was looking good."

My brother Mark followed Bernie's legacy and became a firefighter in the Cleveland system. His training as a paramedic was invaluable. He was always at-the-ready to help as well. Mark made sure she made her appointments and would stop and visit, even after one of his twenty four hour shifts.

Mom moved into an assisted living facility, which was quite nice. She had her own two-bedroom apartment and acquired some new and quality friends. Still driving, she was happy and, critical to her and us, was independent. Mark painted the apartment peach, her favorite color. While it made the place look like a fruit bowl, she loved it. Along with her Cleveland Indians tee-shirt, she was the "Queen of Assisted Living."

We all knew it was going to happen, that time would knock on her door. And it did; gently at first, then with ever-increasing conviction. She began to fall, how often only she knew, but certainly more than she was telling us. The first casualty was a direct hit to her independence; the growing loss of balance forced us to take her car away. Eventually one of the falls broke her hip. She was ninety and the surgeon decided not to put in an artificial hip, only to pin it. A period of uncertainty followed. We didn't know if she would ever walk again. She was determined, though, to return to the assisted living facility where the familiarity of her home and new friends awaited. As is common, a negotiation took place. She could return but one more fall meant an extended care facility. Then, within twenty-four hours of discharge, she admitted she couldn't do it.

My amazingly capable and resourceful sister once again worked her magic and found a newly opened extended care facility within a mile of her former residence. Mom was not happy, instinctively realizing this is where she would be spending her remaining days. Again, neither my siblings nor I extended an invitation to live with one of us. Gawande in *Being Mortal*, points out that where once it was commonplace for the aging parents to live out their final days in the home of one or more of the children—and frequently that still is the case in many other countries— the more westernized a society becomes the more likely the parents will end up in an extended care facility.

I tried to get to Cleveland as much as possible to spend a weekend with her. We even went to a couple of Cleveland Indians games, with baseball and the Indians serving as a familiar anchor in her life. During the visits we had blunt but beneficial conversations about her end of life, and what she wanted. Mom developed a terrible problem with dry mouth; swallowing food was difficult. Finally, it reached a point where she couldn't swallow at all. She was in complete control of her mental faculties and understood everything I told her, and I told her if she stopped eating she would die in two weeks. The alternative was a feeding tube; it was her decision and she was capable of making it. She elected the feeding tube. But that did not add "life to her years."

This was November. My wife, sons, and dog all went to see her. She acknowledged this would be her last Christmas. My mother loved Christmas; loved decorating the Christmas tree, and made an angel affectionately named "Angie". She would make new dresses for Angie as the others deteriorated. I should have brought her to Michigan and our home for that last Christmas even though she would need private nursing and was incontinent of both urine and stool, but I did not make the effort. She died about six weeks later, and I still feel the guilt to this day.

Reviewing the final days of my parents and my wife's mother, my mother had the best end of life, although I didn't feel the feeding tube added any "life to her years." My father had a quality exit, not a lot of medical problems but severe dementia. He didn't die at home, but wouldn't have known it anyway. My wife's mother did not have what I could call quality end of life experiences, but at least her mother got the hot dog and Margarita.

The thoughts above reflect my view of the world. That world, you may have already surmised, is governed by respect for human dignity. Further, Dr. Stein's astute observation regarding "Life to Years versus Years to Life" is never far from my approach to end-of-life decisions. I initiate the discussion regarding end of life dynamics early in my relationship with heart failure patients. I bluntly—but hopefully with some modicum of tact—inform my patients they will enjoy a period of stability followed by a decline, sometimes rapid, where previously effective medication becomes ineffective.

There are alternatives: a continuous infusion of powerful drugs, a Left Ventricular Assist Device (LVAD), a transplant. But the overriding question becomes, "What expectations do you, the patient, have? Depending on the severity of your condition, do you want to do whatever is necessary to be with your family for one more Christmas? Alternatively, do you want to say, "Let nature take its course? I don't want their final memories of me to be as an infirmed onlooker, lacking the strength or ability to participate in the family festivities." I also tell them that hospice has been a truly wonderful alternative. My gratitude is wide and deep for the manner in which the nurses care for my patients and do so while preserving their dignity.

I urge my patients; do not slide into the incoherence of end of life without having presented your wishes to family or physician. If you choose to have everything done, all the resources of medicine brought to bear, then say so. Those resources can add "Years to your Life. But if you see little need for extending the inevitable and want to control your final days and ensure your dignity is preserved, then make your wishes known. While your physician can provide a realistic assessment of your physical condition, your family must assume responsibility for your dignity."

As I write this I am seventy years old. I lead a full life that includes an abundance of challenging physical activity, mostly skiing and the grueling sport of long-distance cycling. My mental acuity is still sharp. But on a clear day I can see that final curtain.

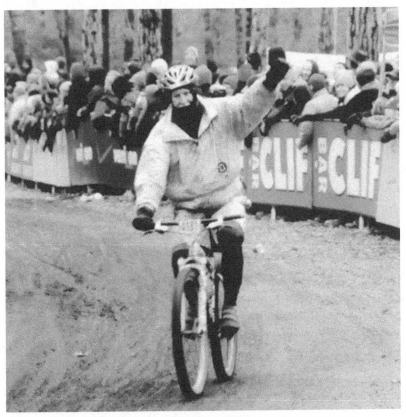

Crossing the finish line. 17 started, 9 finished—I was number 9.
That's a top-ten finish. Mission accomplished.

I have two sons who are physicians, a daughter who is a physical therapist, and my wife is an x-ray technician and a cardiovascular technician. I've always believed that God designed our body to get through the first sixty years, after that its fix-it time. At the insistence of my wife, I recently purchased long-term insurance. While I don't have any major medical problems, aches and pains occasionally invite themselves in for an evening, just to make sure I don't start thinking seventy is the new forty.

I want nothing to do with assisted living, nursing homes, or extended care facilities. My carefully constructed game plan calls for asking the Lord's forgiveness when the "heart rate meter" hits single digits, savoring one more bottle of wine, enjoying one last sexual encounter, and then passing from this world with dignity far from any hospital. I love my other home situated on the shore of the crystal-clear waters of Torch Lake in Bellaire, Michigan. On many occasions, I have uttered the definitive statement that is to govern my own final day: "Give me a bottle of Tequila, and set me adrift in a Viking Boat on Torch Lake with an appropriate dose of Succinylcholine[1], so I can't change my mind at the last minute." We'll see just how flamboyant my final act is when the time comes. And I hope that my actions will prompt somebody to rise at my funeral and say, "He added life to years." What physician could ask for more?

Our progress in caring for heart patients has been nothing short of astounding. We have seen more advancement in the past fifty years than in the previous five thousand years. We can stent arteries, even replace them. We can replace the heart's intricate electrical system and correct abnormal rhythms. We can replace valves. We can replace the entire heart with another. All of which would astound cardiologists and their patients of even a generation ago. We are no longer preserving a community of television watchers. We are succeeding in the noble mission of adding 'Life to Years."

---

1   Succinylcholine is a medication used to induce muscle relaxation and short-term paralysis to assist with tracheal intubation. It also combines with pain medication and sedatives for euthanasia.

While we herald the successes of cardiac care, we do not shy from the uncomfortable; when someone says, "That's enough, I don't want any more years added to my life, if life cannot be added to my years." When that time comes, then the inevitable question arises, how many months do I have left, Doctor? That's when I sit back and retell a story that taught me a lesson some thirty years ago:

> I was an Internal Medicine resident at the Chicago Osteopathic Hospital and was taking care of a janitor who had pancreatic cancer and was not doing well. When he asked me this question, I put my arm around his shoulder and looked him in the eye and said probably less than six months. I moved on and returned to Chicago as a guest lecturer 10 years later and as I was walking toward the auditorium to address the students, I heard a voice behind me say "Hey doc, remember me? Don't ever tell someone that they have six months to live because I will be around to pee on your grave."

Since that day when the inevitable question arises I say only the man upstairs can give you that answer. We have done everything possible to add life to your years so from now on remember, "Every day is a holiday, and every meal is a banquet." And the first part of my lecture that day was to tell the medical students that very story to help them answer that question when posed to them as they progressed through their education.

"Take Me Out..." and "Just a splash of ginger ale— but just a splash..."

We cannot leave our discussion on end of life decisions without telling the amazing stories of Ed Hardin and Harry Bell. They never knew each other and didn't travel in the same circles. But we feel certain they would have liked each other. Both lives were driven by accomplishment, love of family and, most of all, personal dignity.

Dr. Michael James:

While I'm sure I have a reputation for being forthright with patients, and that sometimes translates into insensitivity or harshness, it would be a mistake to assume that I shut off the "I Care" spigot when dealing with terminally ill patients. In that regard, I cannot have an end-of-life discussion without recounting the story of my good friend Ed Harden.

One Sunday morning at seven o'clock I received a phone call informing me that Ed Harden was having difficulty. The assumption was that the name would get my attention and justify waking me at the untimely hour. While I knew Ed Harden was the interim President of Michigan State University, I had no idea why the call was directed my way instead of the cardiologist on duty. I curtly told the caller I shouldn't be bothered with this on an early Sunday morning and hung up. Later, reading the Sunday paper, I learned Ed Harden would be presiding over graduation ceremonies the following Saturday. Being President of Michigan State University would be a big deal anywhere but approaches being royalty in the Lansing/East Lansing area. I immediately contacted the seven o'clock caller and instructed him to have President Harden in my office first thing next morning. I later discovered President Harden wanted me to treat him because I was a DO; he had a special fondness for osteopaths.

The next morning he was at my office at the appointed time. He was short of breath, had a heart rate of 130 and was out of rhythm. I assured him this was all fixable. We would start oral medications to slow his heart rate and I would make daily calls to his office during the upcoming week, carefully monitoring his heart rate. All went well. On Friday I snuck him into the hospital, shocked his heart and off he went to graduation the next day. Outside the hospital a sea of reporters awaited me with questions on President Harden's medical condition. While I toyed with the notion of having some fun and answering the questions in a flip and irreverent manner, thankfully common sense stepped in and seized control. No matter how humorous I thought I was, this was the President of Michigan State University. I provided brief answers that respected President Harden's privacy but assured all that he was medically fit. After I got to know him better I'm confident he would have appreciated the irreverent humor, but at least on this day decorum prevailed.

Ed Harden, I learned, was a troubadour from another time, one of the most capable, interesting, and humble people I have ever known. He is not easily defined. His extensive professional talents were admired by many. Yet he was essentially a very private man. He was the wise and avuncular friend who dispensed counsel on living life to the fullest with great care and precision, yet he reserved the gift of his personal experiences for those closest to him. He carried himself with a sense of detached pride yet he was a genuinely funny man. I felt privileged when he allowed that side of himself to surface during our visits. Ed Harden was a proud man, dignity a driving force in his life becoming even more significant when illness and age converged to rob him of his physical strength. He lived in fear of a stroke that would leave him dependent on others, an unacceptable existence. In the event of a stroke, he instructed, "Take me out." It was not a request, rather a directive he returned to on many occasions. Caught up in the moment and not fully realizing the consequences, I said I would.

Apart from the presidency of two major universities, Ed Harden also served as Chairman of the Board for StoryCorp. StoryCorp is an organization designed to preserve and share humanity's stories and build strong bonds between generations, all designed to create a more just and compassionate world. Through the years, luminaries from the world of government, education, journalism, entertainment and business have served on StoryCorp's prestigious Board of Directors.

Ed Harden knew President Ronald Reagan personally and was extended an invitation by the President himself to visit the White House. Rumors persist to this day that he was offered a cabinet post in the Reagan administration. While Ed's daughter, Pam, doesn't believe so, the rumors remain alive and well. Even Pam admits her dad was a private man and likely would not have made public such an offer.

He invited me to dinner and offered valuable counsel on how to live life as a successful person. He told me on numerous occasions, "Be nice to the little people on the way up, because the trip down can be awfully bumpy." Certainly the observation was not original to him, but it took on a new and indelible meaning when expressed by Ed Harden, especially when it was couched in his ongoing tutorial on handling success.

He gave me his MSU basketball tickets. Far more than just a gratuitous gesture, this was the storybook season of 1979. Earvin "Magic" Johnson and the Spartans were on an exciting and historic journey to the NCAA national Championship. I got to watch every home game from the President's seats.

Ultimately, Ed Harden did have a stroke and was placed in a long-term care facility. I took care of him until he died in his eighties. I regularly visited him on Friday afternoons, always with a chilled Gin Martini escorted by two essential olives. Forbidden as it was, the martini did wonders for his morale. The visits were not easy. Before me was a man of rare achievement, a man I had personally grown very fond of, a man whose professional and personal fingerprints could be found on many lives, mine included. But this productive and active life had been reduced to what could be displayed on the walls of a small room in a long-term care facility. We spoke of many things during those visits but returned repeatedly to living life to its fullest. Because of Ed Harden, whenever patients ask me how best to live their lives, I instinctively recite the advice of my friend, "Every day a holiday, every meal a banquet." With Ed's counsel firmly planted in my own life, I try to do likewise—because you never know when you will wake up peeing blood, and your life has changed forever.

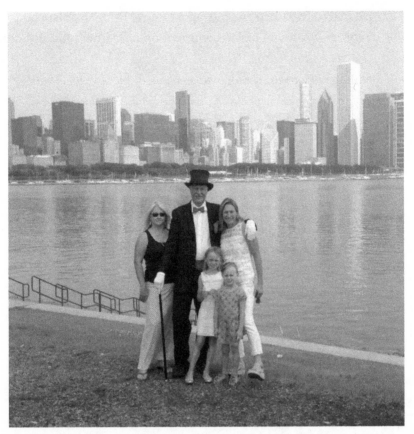

Doing the windy city they way it should be done. Everyday a holiday, every meal a banquet.

During my Friday visits Ed would point his finger and admonish me to keep the promise to "Take me out." I wrestled with Ed's reminder, concluding only that Dr. Jack Kevorkian should not be easily dismissed. I purchased a book titled The Final Exit that gives the precise dose of medications that would accomplish his wish. I seriously considered it. "Take me out" began to occupy more of our Friday afternoon martini dialogues, but having sworn the Hippocratic Oath and being Catholic, I could not do it. Ed was dying, the resolute presence of his pride the only visible remnant of a remarkable life. But I am not God, I told myself. It's not up to me to say who lives and who dies.

My visits were rewarded by getting to know Pam Nyquist, Ed's very capable daughter. We asked her to comment on her father's life and death:

> *"If ever a person was ill prepared emotionally for old age, it was my dad. He never expected to become an eighty-nine-year-old man, convinced I'm sure he would likely die at his desk.*

> *"Work was his life. He rarely took a vacation. I'm confident he fully anticipated his ongoing drive for accomplishment would one-day result in a heart attack. But he could not, would not, ever conceive of a stroke. A stroke was bereft of personal dignity, too horrific for even the most remote of his thoughts.*

> *"Mike James went beyond providing medical support for my father. They respected each other and, not surprisingly, became warm friends. Mike James was blunt—Dad liked and respected that side of him. One reason Mike stood apart from others is he didn't coddle him. The affinity each felt for the other was genuine. Mike's support, along with the love of our family and many close friends and colleagues, was vital to Dad during those final days.*

> *"Ed Harden certainly had his adversaries; you don't live the full life he did without drawing a few penalties along the way. However, the decisiveness that might have alienated some was the very quality in Dad that Mike admired so much. In that regard, the two of them were very much alike. It was easy to understand why Dad welcomed their visits.*

> *"As time went on, I grew closer to Mike James. As he was with Dad, Dr. James was blunt with me about the deteriorating condition. And like Dad, I appreciated that bluntness. We talked a number of times about the promise to "Take me out." Mike had*

a problem with it; not so much filling Dad's final request, but the requirement that he be forced to play God in the process.

"To witness life slowly drain from him tore me up, as it did Mike James. Dad was a man who gave commands not followed them. But this man of many commands now needed assistance for such menial personal tasks as using the bathroom. As his life left him, his frustration and anger mounted.

"Early one morning I got an urgent call from the facility telling me I should come immediately. Walking into the room I asked, "What's going on?"

"He responded, "Just let me go." Dad was eighty-nine years old. He died peacefully; his heart just gave out. I thought about many things that day.

"I thought about the special relationship with Dr. Mike James that not only kept him alive, but more importantly enabled Dad to retain his dignity during the difficult times. Years before Dad developed a special affinity for doctors of osteopathy. As an administrator at the university, he engineered the transfer of the College of Osteopathy from Pontiac to Michigan State University, where it remains to this day. He worked on their behalf most of his life. Dad was once asked if he would like a second opinion regarding his treatment, namely the Mayo Clinic and/or the Cleveland Clinic, both highly acclaimed for their treatment of heart patients. He would have none of it – Mike James was one of the best; he didn't need to go anywhere else.

"I thought about Dad's career. He served as president of two universities, Northern Michigan University and Michigan State University. His tenure as President of Michigan State University was the crowning moment of a truly extraordinary professional life. Dad loved politics, loved being able to move the frequently sluggish machinery of the political system for the common good. While he was neither a Republican nor Democrat, such was his understanding of politics I am convinced he would have made an outstanding governor.

"I thought about Dad's truly remarkable life. He grew up in a railroad-and-farm town in Iowa and eloped with his high school sweetheart. They had a rich and long married life together. He went to college on a baseball scholarship, a left-hander who played first base. He was good, too, at one point attracting interest from some major league teams.

"And I thought about the fact that he was my dad, and how much he gave me as a parent. I thought about the love he had for my brother and how proud he was of him, and of their shared interests and accomplishments.

"I thought about how many lives he had touched, and how very fortunate our family had been to know such a caring, devoted, and loyal physician as Mike James to help us along the painful path."

Mike Ranville:

"The greatest dignity to be found in death is the dignity of the life that preceded it."
—ANONYMOUS

Harry Bell defied labels; he was not easily slotted.

Shakespeare wrote, "All the world's a stage, and all the men and women merely players; they have their exits and their entrances; and one man in his time plays many parts."[2]

When Harry died at 97 on April 22, 2016, the many roles he played in life were summoned to tell his amazing story and deployed to fashion an extraordinary epitaph. Significantly, dignity was central to each of the roles. Dignity governed Harry's life and ultimately his death.

On February 19, 1942, a little more than two months after the beginning of World War II, 24-year-old Harry Bell was cast in the role of a soldier and enlisted in the Army Air Corps. He mastered the art of a waist gunner and flew many missions in the European theater on a B-17 christened the "Millie K."

On September 28, 1944, the "Millie K" was hit by flak forcing the crew to bail out over Germany. Harry and his fellow crew members were captured and sent to a POW camp in Poland—Stalag Luft IV. He escaped but was re-captured. The escape embarrassed his captors; there was hell to pay when the Germans caught him. Along with his fellow escapees, he was beaten—according to his daughter Sherry, "beaten real bad." Harry firmly believed they intended to beat them all to death. He credits survival to one of his buddies who could speak Polish and passable German, and that appeared to strike a chord of humanity in one of the German soldiers. He was returned to Stalag Luft IV where he remained for the next eight months.

In early 1945, following their breakout at Stalingrad, Soviet forces began to advance rapidly, forcing the Germans to abandon Stalag Luft IV. On February 6, 1945, during one of the most severe winters in European history, 6,000 American and British POWs—Staff Sergeant Harry Bell among them—were roused without notice to set out on a 600-mile forced march across Northern Germany. While not as well documented, it was every bit the equal of the horrendous Bataan Death March in the Philippines. For 87 days they marched. Conditions were inhumane. There

---

2   Shakespeare, William, *As You Like It,* Act 2, Scene 7.

were no sanitary facilities. The marchers were forced to subsist on 700 calories of food a day[3]—and that's if and when the Germans distributed the Red Cross food parcels. In the midst of sub-zero temperatures, the prisoners had wholly inadequate shoes and clothing.

Disease was rampant, including typhus fever, dysentery, body lice, diphtheria, pneumonia, and pellagra. Frostbite was a major problem, resulting in many crude and unsterile amputations. Frozen ground served as a bed. The men rallied to each other. Harry developed a severe case of tonsillitis. Humor supplanted non-existent medicine. Healthier marchers spent their days carrying the infirmed, and then caring for them at night. Coats were shared. Later, during testimony before the War Crimes Commission, the march was aptly described as a "domain of heroes."

Harry Bell maintains dried onions saved his life. He packed his shirt and pants with the onions for insulation, and those same onions saved him from sure starvation. He would look fondly upon onions for his remaining days. Due to disease, starvation, below-zero temperatures, and being gunned down by German soldiers during escape attempts, 1,500 marchers did not survive. But Harry Bell did. Armed only with his resolute spirit and keen wits, Harry not only survived, he escaped.

Distance from his captors brought no relief from the frigid temperatures. Harry made his way to nearby historic Juterbog, a village in north-eastern Germany about 65 miles south-west of Berlin. He was taken in by a sympathetic German family, grateful to the allies for their efforts in ending the oppression of the Third Reich; so grateful that the man offered Harry his wife.

Harry recalls the gracious hospitality with a wry smile. "I was too sick to take advantage of the offer—not that I would have anyway." After a few days to gather his strength, he stole a bike from a youngster and rode it to the nearby Nuthe River. He waved his hands to the Russians on the other side who rescued him. The Russian Soldiers guided him to

---

3   POWs under U.S. jurisdiction received 3,500 calories per day.

the American lines. He was placed on an American Hospital Ship and eventually recuperated at the Veterans Hospital in Battle Creek.

Before being honorably separated from military service on December 9, 1945, Staff Sergeant Harry Bell's service to his country was recognized. He was awarded the Purple Heart, the Good Conduct Medal, the American Theater Ribbon, the Air Medal, three bronze campaign stars, European, African, and Middle Eastern Ribbons and the World War II Victory Medal.

Despite the wretched conditions of Stalag Luft IV, the near death beating after an escape, and the 600 mile march across Northern Germany in sub-zero weather, Harry Bell returned to Michigan and the love of his life, Marjorie Fairchild—dignity intact. Within a month of his separation from active duty, he married Marjorie and settled comfortably into the role of husband, the union lasting 65 years until her death in 2011. They settled in Charlotte, Michigan, where he became something of a local legend.

During the next few years he spent considerable time learning new roles. He sold his 1948 Harley Davidson and built a house. His part was re-written to accommodate four children; his performance was outstanding. He went to work for the Eaton County Road Commission where he was cast in the role of a foreman. It fit well; ended up playing it for thirty years.

Harry's daughter Sherry described her father as, "down-to-earth, the kind of guy you just want to have a beer with"—and as it turned out, many would lay claim to doing just that. His drink of preference, though, was whiskey, water and ginger ale—"but just a splash of ginger ale." That drink of preference became an integral part of the Harry Bell legend.

Harry was a people magnet. Sherry tells how their home was constant activity. "We had lots of company," she says. "Sometimes they would just talk or play cards. But there was always laughing—and a couple of toddies of course." Harry was a genuinely funny man, possessor of a lightening wit. One of his VFW buddies described him as a "One-man USO show." And he was no slave to political correctness. "He was perpetual flirt," she says; "called all the ladies 'honey' and he got away with it."

The gruff exterior could not hide the warmth inside. The neighborhood children loved him. His kibitzing was accompanied by a twinkle that never left his eye. And when the summer days warmed he was a soft touch for an ice cream bar. Sherry recalls the time when a youngster was visiting with his parents. The young man mentioned his dog in the conversation, and that the dog was not doing well. Months later when Harry encountered the young man, he quickly asked, "How's that dog of yours?"

He loved his family. In addition to his own children, he was particularly close to his granddaughter Michelle and her husband Barry. He beamed when his great-granddaughter Breanna was around, and that was often. They called him "Papa." Breanna and Papa would talk – about everything. She looked to him for counsel, and he didn't disappoint. He would tell her, "You don't have to make every decision today. You're young. Be happy."

Breanna tells a story that captures the essence of her great-grandfather. The two were at a wedding and the Reverend was going on interminably with what was supposed to be a short grace before the meal. Harry, in a bellowing whisper, said to Breanna, "If he doesn't quit praying we're never going to get a drink."

"He went through hell during World War II," Sherry observed, "and he came out a decent man—I don't know how."

Like many returning veterans who had seen more than their share of combat, Harry rarely talked about his war experiences. Not long after he came home he did recount one or two events. People looked at him in disbelief, suggesting he was embellishing his war record in an attempt to draw attention to himself. "He didn't need to lie about his record," Sherry says, "his story stands on its own." Fearing people would not believe him he stopped talking about his war experiences altogether.

"Mom didn't like the war stories and would get real aggravated when he told one,' Sherry recalls, "so he didn't talk about the war." After Marjorie died—five years nearly to the day before Harry died—Sherry and the other family members said to him, "Dad, how are we going to know if you don't tell us? How's anyone going to know what you went through? Your family and friends need to know that side of you."

Harry started talking, gradually at first, but enough to let his family know of the ordeal. His buddies at the VFW had stories of their own. That helped immensely.

For the record, Harry's granddaughter Michelle points out, "After he started talking about his experiences, the stories never wavered. There was no embellishing or changing the facts to make him sound like a hero. It was always the same story, hardly the way a self-serving impostor would go about it."

Harry enjoyed life in Charlotte, Michigan. He was surrounded by family and a solid core of friends. He bought land around Houghton Lake, and built a cabin on it with his own hands. There was a house ready for demolition in nearby Vermontville. Harry tore it down himself and used the lumber to build the place at Houghton Lake. While the cabin would never get beyond rustic, he loved it. It had all he wanted in life; family and friends—and, of course, whiskey and water with just a splash of ginger ale—but just a splash.

For his greatest battle Harry summoned the dignity that hovered over him all his life, especially during the war. His final role may have been his saddest, but it was his finest. And, as always, he was at his best when performing with long-time co-star and loyal companion, his dignity.

The near starvation he endured during the 600 mile march across Northern Germany left its mark. During his later years he was forced to wear a colostomy bag. Wearing it was bad enough, but one day it broke. While Harry shooed everyone away, Sherry came over and cleaned it up. Harry didn't see it as an accident, rather as a sign people would now have to take care of him. His self-esteem, not the colostomy, was the issue.

Harry had heart problems, had trouble breathing, and sought treatment from the Thoracic Cardiovascular Institute, the famed TCI group of cardiologists. His cardiologist was none other than Dr. Mike James. Harry and Dr. James were fond of each other. Harry liked the doctor's blunt approach. "If there was something wrong, he would tell you, and wouldn't sugar-coat it," Harry confided to his daughter.

At one point Harry got tangled up when he tried to take the dog out. The family found him on the floor his head covered in blood. He wouldn't wear a life support button. When the nurse came to visit him he was embarrassed, called himself a "dummy." The family decided he needed someone with him 24-7. They worked in shifts.

The quality of his life was deteriorating. Harry was a tinkerer, always finding something to do. But the time came when he couldn't tinker anymore. "I can do the projects in my mind," he would say, "but my body just won't get up and do them." Harry loved riding around town with his dog Blackie, waving to friends while nursing a *whiskey and water with just a splash of ginger ale, but just a splash.* But now he couldn't drive anymore.

He was diagnosed with Atrial Fibrillation, where the top and bottom chambers of the heart do not beat in sync. He underwent cardioversion, where an electrical impulse is sent to the heart to shock both chambers into synchronization. It worked at first, but the breathing problems returned. Dr. James told him the A-Fib was not a death sentence, but he had to slow down. Three weeks before he died, Harry took a turn for the worse and developed congestive heart failure. Dr. James told Harry there was nothing more he could do. His heart was going to tick until it stopped ticking. Harry responded, "I'm ready for it to stop ticking." Harry knew his time was near, and he was ready. His wife's ashes were beside his chair and he would talk to her. "Okay, Ma. I'm coming. I'm ready."

Harry Bell told all that he was ready. His dignity was undergoing a daily assault. Dr. James suggested Hospice be brought in; Harry agreed. He knew precisely what Hospice was and what it meant. He even helped fill out the paperwork. The Hospice nurses loved him. His only reservation—and he was adamant about it—he did not want to go to any facility; he wanted to die at home. Sherry assured him no facility.

He had complete control of his mental faculties, right up to the very end. Two nights before he died he was visiting with friends—laughing, joking, trading barbs—he knew exactly who they were. His final concern was his dog Blackie; who would take care of him? Blackie was a Chihuahua, found in a dumpster in Tennessee. The bond between Harry and Blackie was unassailable. Blackie now lives in comfort with Sherry.

A month after he died the life of Harry Bell was celebrated at the Charlotte VFW Post 2406. It was a packed house. The program was equal parts tears and laughter. The bar was kept busy that day serving an inordinate number of *whiskey and waters with just a splash of ginger ale— but just a splash.* Taps were sounded. Salutes were rendered. Harry Bell was laid to rest—dignity intact.

In recognition of the extraordinary service to his country, on September 29, 2016, former Staff Sergeant Harry Bell was laid to rest - at Arlington National Cemetery.

CHAPTER TWO:

The Journey Begins

"Wherever the art of medicine is loved, there is also a love of humanity."
—HIPPOCRATES

Dr. Michael James:

For as long as I can remember, I was going to be a doctor. At first I thought it was because my dad, Bernie James, told me so when I was still in kindergarten. Bernie's ability to influence a decision was not lightly discarded. But I quickly warmed to the idea, especially after announcing my decision to a nun at school. From then on, at least in her eyes, this kindergartener could do no wrong. Apparently for her, medicine ranked just below the priesthood as a chosen career. In any event, I never looked back.

Bernie James had an angular, chiseled appearance. While he was slow to smile, the playful twinkle was never far from the surface. The eyes spoke volumes. They bored in on you, leaving the impression that he always knew more than he was saying, and he did. They commanded attention and respect; he was not easily dismissed. And they were an amazing window to the world for those of us around him. He was a man of purpose and experience and it seemed he always had one more resource to draw on to solve a problem.

Dad's effort to steer me into medicine was understandable. He was a medic in the Army; not your ordinary medic but an RKG technician. I always suspected he yearned to be a doctor but his father left the family at an early age and as the eldest he assumed responsibility for a younger brother and sister.

After the war he earned a college degree under the GI Bill and eventually became a firefighter, a career destination for most, but not for Dad. He decided to go to law school, attended classes at night. For years the fireman/lawyer was the attorney of choice for his fellow firefighters. He even kept a phone in his locker at the firehouse and would answer as if it was his law office. He retired as a firefighter and attorney.

Once after a day of golf, we were coming out of a bar with a six-pack of long-necks in tow. Waiting for us at our car were a couple of thugs who demanded his wallet—or else. Without hesitation, he threw the six-pack on the ground, took a bottle in each hand, and broke them on the cement. Brandishing the jagged-edged bottles, he told the thugs to stand aside or someone was going to the hospital, and it wouldn't be him. They quickly discerned Dad was not someone to trifle with; intuition told me this was not his maiden voyage dealing with street punks.

On another occasion when he was in law school, there were those who sought to take advantage of this lawyer/fireman. They invited him to a poker game. He came home, hung over, after losing big time. According to him, the boys just kept buying him beers. The following week he came home after the poker game and threw a pocketful of money on the kitchen table.

"How did you do it?" I asked.

He laughed and told me every time they bought him a beer he would go in the men's room, pour the beer out, and then fill the bottle with water. He put on a drunken act and instead of donating to the cause ended up taking their money.

But there was more to Bernie James than the street smart, wily poker player. He convinced two of my friends not to go to work at the local General Motors plant after high school. He lent both college tuition money, and both rewarded him by graduating. To friends and acquaintances Bernie James was a forceful, dynamic presence. By no means a saint, he lived life with a certain swagger that I absolutely adored. I cannot overstate the influence Dad had on my life, both personally and professionally. I am not only a better doctor because of him, but a better person as well.

My mother affectionately nicknamed "Mame" was the glue that kept the family together. She was an excellent seamstress and made most of our clothes. She was a wonderful cook that could make pork and sauerkraut, pierogies, galumkis—all that great ethnic food. Most of all, she was a devout Catholic who went to Mass every Sunday and prayed that her offspring would be successful.

While I was not a member of MENSA, I got good grades, primarily because I possessed a stubborn work ethic and a strong sense of competition. My approach to life could be equated to the constant, unremitting journey of the mill stone that grinds the wheat. Like the mill stone I am a "grinder," not the most sophisticated of tools, but one that will never be outworked. When Dad's tenacity genes were added to the equation, this grinder could proudly stand on equal ground with the gifted. Still, medical school seemed an impossibly high bar. But that grinder mentality served me well in college and medical school and has remained a welcome and influential companion throughout my life.

In that regard, my brother became a firefighter and a paramedic. My sister, a teacher; she continues to work supervising and evaluating would be teachers at Nazareth College in Cleveland, Ohio. Bernie James's presence in our lives was never far from the surface.

Born and raised in Cleveland, Ohio, I am the product of a Jesuit education. The nuns suggested I skip the seventh grade and head directly into the eighth. While I was not in favor of the move, Dad thought it a good idea, so I became an eighth grader.

Like many young lads of my age I was interested in sports. But skinny kids who tip the scale at 105 pounds, and are the youngest in their class, don't get taken seriously on the playing fields. My athletic career at St.

Ignatius High School never caught traction. The alternative was to channel my energy into becoming a good student.

After high school I determined success in life hinged on the right college and I applied at both Notre Dame and Georgetown. However, I didn't do well with the college-board exam. Wrestling with standardized admission tests would haunt me throughout my life.

I eventually attended the University of Detroit, a fine Jesuit school, and graduated in the top 25 percent of my class. With a solid credential of academic accomplishment, I assumed the medical school of my choice awaited; just mail in the application, the only concern being the roommate I would draw. But I did not do well on the standardized Medical College Admission Test (MCAT) and was turned away wherever I applied, without fail a low score on the test cited as the reason.

Disappointed and angry, I enlisted the President of the University of Detroit to intercede on my behalf, stressing that I was a top student with a resume that included a number of worthwhile extra-curricular activities.

Nothing.

Some of my classmates were in the same position and decided to apply to the Chicago College of Osteopathy. What was Osteopathy? In Michigan, osteopathic physicians were accepted as primary care providers with an emphasis on the musculoskeletal system. However, unlike chiropractors, they also believed in pharmaceutical preparations and surgery. I applied and was accepted, but quickly discovered the stigma attached to osteopathy; 90 percent of my class would rather have been starting their training in a medical school as opposed to a school for doctors of osteopathy.

Initially I was wary. I learned in Illinois doctors of osteopathy did not enjoy full practice rights. In fact, both the Dean and Chief of Surgery went back to Northwestern and earned MD degrees so they could sign off on prescriptions and surgical reports, a privilege not accorded DOs at the time.

The Chicago College of Osteopathy was located in Hyde Park, Illinois, close to the prestigious University of Chicago. Although there was no official affiliation, we were welcome to attend various seminars and conferences. While my basic medical education was acquired at the Chicago College of Osteopathy, some of the more formative education was from the University of Chicago.

When I started my Internal Medicine residency, I wanted a challenge and I wanted diversity. I insisted on spending time at all seven of the Chicago medical schools. This meant going head-to-head with MDs; the competitor in me relished the opportunity. The grinder surfaced – and seized control.

I vowed early on no one was going to outwork me; further, that my medical career would be driven by old-fashioned common sense. The MDs had the same text-books we had; they put their pants on one leg at a time as we did. The only difference between them and us was the score on a standardized test. I refused to be intimidated.

At that time, I embraced what would become a steadfast rule of my medical practice: trust yourself 100 percent of the time, and your mother 50 percent of the time, and no one else, ever. That philosophy has never failed me.

I also adopted another rule, equally as important; be frank and honest with patients. Unfortunately, many of my colleagues don't subscribe to that theory and are reluctant to convey anything but good news. They practice "lawsuit medicine"[4], where the truth can become a casualty. Conversely, I became a strong proponent of including patients in their care. They have a right to be involved in decisions that impact their lives; they deserve our candor as well as our medical expertise.

Osteopathy school was coming to an end. I needed to choose a career path. I instinctively knew that you cannot treat what you cannot diagnose, and you cannot diagnose what you don't know. Many of my classmates sought me out for help in explaining EKG (Electrocardiogram) results. Perhaps I had a facility for cardiology. Moreover, heart disease was still the number one killer in the United States. This newly-minted member

---

4   For the record, I have been practicing medicine since 1969. Only one lawsuit has ever been filed against me, and that was thrown out for lack of a credible witness for the plaintiff.

of the medical profession was intrigued with improving the quality of life for heart patients.

Thinking back, the attraction to cardiology was understandable. It was logical; the challenge was never in the diagnosis but in the treatment. The heart is really very simple – valves, muscles, arteries, electrical system, that's it. And to my inquisitive black-and-white, never-gray, mind, it made sense. I was also drawn by the rapid pace of growth in cardiac technology. I sensed—accurately as it turns out—that the explosion of research involving the heart would render a career in cardiology exciting and rewarding.

The lure of home and Cleveland was largely responsible for my accepting an internship in nearby Cuyahoga Falls, Ohio. But the basic question remained—how to secure a Fellowship with my osteopathic training?

After my general internship in Ohio, I returned to Chicago, the carrot being if I would agree to teach, the college would sponsor me for further training in cardiology. The Chief of Medicine at the Chicago College of Osteopathy, Ward Perrin III, explained that if DOs were ever going to be relevant as a profession, a complete education was needed. If I would make a two-year teaching commitment to the Chicago College of Osteopathy, I could go anywhere that would accept me for a Fellowship.

At that time Park Willis at the University of Michigan felt that as a public institution, there was an inherent obligation to serve the state of Michigan. He pointed out there were many DOs practicing in the state and if they agreed to train me I would, in turn, be obligated to teach others. I quickly agreed.

I was accepted at the University of Michigan for my Cardiology Fellowship, thrown in with five highly recruited MD's for the two-year program. They were chosen; I came in through the "back door." My old friend the grinder surfaced. As always, he refused to sit in the back of the class. The plan was simple; read more, prepare more, work harder.

I loved my time in Ann Arbor. It was that special era in the storied football rivalry between the University of Michigan and Ohio State

University, the over-hyped annual battle between Bo Schembechler and Woody Hayes. As part of the Fellowship, I was on the Cardiac Arrest Team at "The Big House" (Michigan Stadium) for Saturday afternoon home games. In those days, unbelievable as it seems, anyone could bring as much alcohol as they wanted into the stadium. In the student section, pony kegs were even allowed. In addition to handling cardiac arrests, we also cared for the large number of intoxicated fans.

Life was good. It was 1972 and I was at the University of Michigan for a two-year fellowship in cardiology. Those were productive years, both for the field of cardiac care and me personally. We expanded the public education effort to stress the importance of getting the patient to a hospital as soon as heart attack symptoms were discerned, action that was paramount to survival. Those public education programs had a positive influence. Citizen training in CPR significantly increased. The greater Seattle, Washington, area boasted that 70 percent of its citizens were trained in CPR. There was compelling evidence of a correlation between citizen training and the saving of lives. Prior to our efforts, in the event of cardiac arrest outside the hospital, the chances of getting to the hospital alive and returning home without sustaining permanent neurological damage was approximately 5 percent. That figure dramatically improved with the advent of Automatic External Defibrillators (AEDs).

We also worked on "blind defibrillation." If an EKG was not available when the Cardiac Arrest Team arrived on the scene, the new directive was to defibrillate immediately. "Blind Defibrillation" was rooted in the knowledge that if circulation to the brain was not restored in four minutes from the onset of a heart attack, permanent neurological damage would likely result.

From a personal standpoint I was proud and enthused to be a part of the University of Michigan cardiac program, acknowledged as one of the world's finest. I arrived there by way of sponsorship by the College of Osteopathic Medicine in Chicago. My mission was clear—I was to secure the best possible training and then return to Chicago where I would teach medical students and strengthen the educational program for the Osteopathic profession.

U of M did it right. Substantively they knew and acknowledged their well-earned sterling reputation. But they had style as well, and I absolutely loved it. They wrapped our introduction to the program in a cloak of University of Michigan folklore. One day one all new staff gathered in an auditorium. We were escorted to our seats by "The Victors," the legendary U of M fight song. Several faculty members were adorned in their Block M or Maize and Blue blazers. We were informed of the distinct and unique honor we now enjoyed; to be called a "Michigan Man" or "Michigan Woman."[5] Wherever we went in the world we would encounter Michigan graduates doing great things. Following the "you have been carefully chosen" speech, we would have marched through walls.

My personal exhilaration was enhanced by the fact that I was only the second DO ever to be accepted into the vaunted cardiac program. This grinder, who had labored long into many nights, was now sitting as an equal alongside those who had been plucked from the very top of their prestigious medical schools. I vowed, as I had throughout the entirety of my academic life, that I would not be outworked.

I immersed myself into the University of Michigan. Personally and professionally, life was rewarding.

I made many friends and could not wait to get to work every day. I lived on the Huron River and could bike to the hospital. I played softball, basketball, touch football, and even rugby for the Ann Arbor Academics.

We rented a house from a professor who was on sabbatical at the Stanford Think Tank for a year. At the time we already had two children and my youngest daughter was born at the university hospital. Sadly, the professor's wife passed away during his year at Stanford. It was my second year of fellowship, and instead of moving back to his home, the professor wrote and said because he was now single and we had three children, he would rent an apartment for the next year so we didn't have to move. I was

---

5   While currently the ratio of men and women is 50:50, in my class of sixty-five students only three were women.

grateful. In the midst of the rigorous academic demands that dominated my life, I wouldn't have to undergo the tremendous stress associated with moving my family. While this type of plot only unfolds in sappy movies, I witnessed first-hand a "Michigan Man" looking out for another "Michigan Man." Cue the violins.

The program was everything I expected; demanding, challenging, arduous, but fulfilling beyond what I ever dreamed possible. I loved the subject matter. I knew, was absolutely convinced, I was in the right place.

Not all the knowledge at U of M was acquired within the rigid confines of the cardiology program. Other invaluable lessons, such as making friends with the nurses and treating them with the respect they deserve, were also learned – for me, the hard way.

I was on the night shift and one of the nurses made a suggestion regarding a patient. My response was, "You're just a nurse, "I'm in charge." Big mistake. That exchange occurred at eleven o'clock, right at shift change. I was on call that night, so every hour or so the nurse phoned me, usually just as I was drifting off to sleep. "Doctor, the patient's temperature is 98.6 degrees." I responded that was normal.

"What do I know?" she shot back. "I'm just a nurse." At two o'clock she called with lab results. I told her those were normal.

"What do I know? I'm just a nurse."

The interruptions, accompanied by the now too-familiar acerbic rejoinder, "I'm just a nurse," continued throughout the night. At six o'clock she bluntly informed me, "Look, I know you've had a lot of schooling, but I came up through the school of hard knocks."

I suggested we have a cup of coffee, at which time she let me know that along with other nurses she had been sitting bedside with that patient for twelve hours, and that I could learn from them. She didn't embroider the message. I should regularly consult the entire medical team and if I did, the true beneficiary would be the patient.

From that day on, I always conferred with the nurses, the techs, actually anyone involved with the patient, before making a decision. While she didn't channel Miss Congeniality when delivering her message, that nurse was absolutely right. I always pass this vital piece of information on to my students, residents, and Fellows, along with the story of how I learned it. There's no such thing as just a nurse. Involve the team, especially the nurses. They can bail you out of trouble, or make you look like a fool. More importantly, though, the patient benefits.

Cognizant of my mission on behalf of the Chicago College of Osteopathy, I spent as much time as I could doing extra work and perfecting my skills. I knew when I returned to Chicago my role would be "the go-to guy."

My time in Ann Arbor was drawing to a close. Among the many great memories are those that involved the mandate that the Cardiac Fellows form the Cardiac Arrest Team at Michigan Stadium for home football games. Game days frequently involved running up and down the steps of the Big House when someone had, or was suspected of having, a heart attack.

I was there when the volatile Ohio State University coach Woody Hayes snapped the down markers. While every game day at the Big House was fraught with excitement, this particular Saturday was more emotional than most. I received at least six calls for possible heart attacks. Thankfully none of those calls came from Bo or Woody.

Before leaving the University of Michigan, there was a graduation ceremony. Every finishing Fellow had to say a few words. While most were schmaltzy, not mine. I complained that for the past two years I had to listen to "Hail to the Victors." Now, I told the audience, nobody ever sang the osteopathic version. And I proceeded to rectify that obvious oversight:

"Hippity hoppity Osteopathy, run right down your spine;

Fix the lesion, lateral flex, you will feel just fine.

Yes! Osteopathy!"

My effort earned a standing ovation. Despite the warm reception, I refused to abandon my medical career; show biz would have to wait.

The pride and sense of accomplishment I felt regarding my tenure at the University of Michigan knew no bounds. I was one of only five osteopathic cardiologists in the nation to be fellowship trained. I was ready for the return to Chicago. Such was my elation that I distinctively recall driving over the Chicago Skyway, uncharacteristically shouting at the top of my lungs, "I'm back, Chicago, and I'm going to own you!" As part of that impromptu soliloquy, still in full voice, I recited what I could remember of Carl Sandburg's great poem, Chicago.

"Hog Butchers of the World,

Tool maker, stackers of wheat,

Player with railroads and the nation's freight handlers,

Stormy, husky, brawling,

City of the big shoulders."

My two years in Ann Arbor convinced me I had indeed arrived. I was getting the best training in the world and eagerly anticipated a career of teaching and practicing modern day cardiology. The adrenaline was flowing. But first I needed to fulfill my commitment to Dr. Perrin so I returned to Chicago to teach DOs.

One Saturday morning while I was making rounds, Dr. Perrin sauntered into the hospital and pulled me aside for a private moment. He was having chest pressure and didn't want to bother anyone. I immediately arranged for him to go in the hospital. We soon learned he had incurred a heart attack. He became my patient and underwent successful coronary bypass surgery at a later date.

Dr. Perrin lived in Hyde Park and walked to work every morning, ritually smoking his pipe. He looked and dressed like Sherlock Holmes. I had spent many hours in his office discussing cases as he lit bowl after bowl while critiquing my presentations. Ward Perrin III and Park Willis, I discovered, were very similar in demeanor.

My career choice to teach and practice cardiology was reinforced when I received "Teacher of the Year" two years in a row. My two-year commitment to Dr. Perrin and the Chicago College of Osteopathy fulfilled, I began looking for a place where I could practice and teach cardiology. While I was fond of my job in Chicago, I lived an hour from work and I dreaded, obsessed over, fighting the traffic twice a day.

The frustration became so intense that I would put my emergency lights on and drive on the shoulder. When stopped I indicated I was on call and responding to an emergency. I was stopped so frequently that it became necessary to refine my bearing of false witness. I took to informing Chicago's finest that I was on my way to the hospital where a police officer was having a heart attack. When the same cop stopped me a third time, I was busted. He offered me a police escort to the hospital. I walked into the Emergency Room, staffed with friends, winking, asking where the cop was that had a heart attack. While I won that particular battle, I lost the war. The alibi had worn thin.

Besides the traffic on Lake Shore Drive, the need to move on was underscored by the fact that we had three children, ages six, five, and three. I wanted something more than a wretched daily commute for them.

The Teacher and the Move

I always had a number of students and residents in tow wherever I went. It was challenging, but it was also rewarding. The "Educator of the Year" award meant a great deal to me. But I was also frustrated, and the frustration continued to fester.

I was living in Evanston, an hour commute on the best of days down Lake Shore Drive. I tried riding my bike but that took me through questionable neighborhoods and added precious hours to the commute. The only hospital affiliated with the school at the time was in Hyde Park, greatly restricting where I could practice my craft. While I loved the job, the commute only served to extend my work day to twenty-two hours and became the bane of my existence.

I have always pursued a number of after-work activities, mostly physical; they were essential to maintaining some sort of balance in my life. Now those pursuits were subordinated to work and the dreaded commute. I was concerned that without some interests outside of medicine, the finely honed edge I had always maintained at work would suffer.

There were other frustrations. After all my training, and the personal sacrifices involved in pursuit of that training, I needed to practice medicine where I could treat the entire patient and not have to rely on another institution. I readily admit that control weighed heavy in defining that need. I had invested too much of my life preparing to be a cardiologist to casually relinquish the care of a patient just because someone else had access to more sophisticated and current tools. When your patient requires a procedure or service you cannot provide, you immediately move into the "second fiddle section of the orchestra." I was not content with playing second fiddle. While recognizing there are several members of a cardiac team involved in the care of a patient, I had earned the right and was qualified to "raise the baton and conduct the entire orchestra."

After two years I felt my obligation to the Chicago College of Osteopathy was complete. I had returned to them the same amount of time they had accorded me to study at the University of Michigan. After a great deal of introspection, wrestling with whether or not I had fulfilled my good faith commitment to the University of Michigan to educate osteopaths in cardiology, and then actually undertaking that educational responsibility in Chicago, I began an active search for a job.

I knew Michigan State University had a new Osteopathic School. Due to the influence, hard work, and persistence of a future patient, Ed Harden, the Osteopathic School had just transferred from Pontiac to Michigan State University in East Lansing. The more I learned the more attractive MSU became. Nearby, Ingham Medical Hospital had a cardiac surgical program, a catheterization lab, full-time students, interns, residents, and a Cardiac Fellowship and, of no small significance to me, was located in a town that wasn't gridlocked twice a day by traffic. I was told a big part of the job at MSU was teaching cardiology at the University. Further, I would be able to do clinical work at the rapidly growing cardiac program at Ingham Medical. I loved Michigan and also loved being part of a university community.

Michigan State University, and all the cultural and social accouterments it offered, coupled with working at a progressive hospital like Ingham Medical, presented an ideal career and family environment for me. I was enthused. The opportunity to teach as well as practice cardiology, and do so in an environment not beset with battling the demons of a daily commuter gridlock; it was a dream come true.

While at the University of Michigan I had made the acquaintance of another DO, George Kleiber, who was one year ahead of me. George had a two-year commitment to the Navy and was working at Michigan State University. George was on the faculty at MSU but doing his clinical work at Ingham Medical Center. In addition to George, the staff consisted of three medical doctors and two cardiac surgeons. George instructed the osteopathic medical students in the tenets of cardiology, a ten-week course of intensified lectures. I contacted him, and he paved the way. With his help I was hired by MSU College of Osteopathic Medicine. I left Chicago with fond memories, having truly enjoyed the fruits of big-city living. But I instinctively knew that residing in a small college town would be a great fit.

The benefits could not be ignored. When housing prices were placed alongside those of Chicago, it was nothing short of a bargain. A relaxed drive to and from work could not be overrated; it will never be taken for granted again. The schools for the kids were great. I would be living in the shadow of a major university; big-time college sports, as well as the cultural and entertainment offerings. And last but certainly not least, there was that great cathedral of the outdoors, what Michigan people refer to simply as "up North."

I was busy on the day I arrived and will be busy on the last day I leave, whenever that should occur. While employed by MSU, I worked eight hours per week at the hospital. The structure at MSU was not that rigid so I ended up working four hours a week at the university, the rest at the hospital. George Kleiber and I became the top producers. We were bringing in money, lots of money, money that we never saw. The group, the Dean, the Provost, and everyone else—all were benefiting, everyone but George and me. We decided to quit the University, volunteer to teach, and become full partners in what was known then as the Mid-Michigan Medical Group.

Things went well. I was doing what I was trained to do, what I wanted to do. I became Fellowship Director, Chairman of Cardiology, and

Director of the Catheterization Lab. I found myself on more committees then there was time in the day. Despite drowning in administrative duties, I insisted on continuing to see patients. I have been blessed throughout the years with the opportunity to treat and know some truly fascinating people from all walks of life.

As excited as I was, the first few days were not without some speed bumps. I had to prove myself once again, which meant being monitored in the catheterization lab. My first battle involved the most effective procedure for a catheterization, the arm or the groin, the same battle waged two years earlier at the University of Michigan. At Ingham Medical they were still doing catheterizations from the arm with a cut down to the brachial artery. Resurrecting the same arguments, I pointed out the advantages of using the groin. The cardiologist monitoring me insisted I do at least one procedure utilizing the arm, which I did. After securing full privileges, though, I successfully changed the catheterization lab over to the groin approach, which saved time and money for everyone, including the patient.

I loved the outdoors, northern Michigan in particular. I was on the statewide CPR (Cardio Pulmonary Resuscitation) committee and invited a faculty member from Petoskey—located high up "at the tip of the mitten"—to teach the course with me. In the back of my mind was the thought that maybe Petoskey was a better place to practice. It certainly would save me from driving up north every weekend. I love skiing; all three of our kids were ski racers. We talked and I accepted a position at the Burns Clinic in Petoskey. It only lasted a year. I didn't feel fulfilled without students, residents, and interacting with Fellows.

I returned to Lansing, and resumed where I left off. Our group was expanding and the heart volume was increasing. This was the heyday of cardiac surgery, of cardiac catheterization and cardiac devices. And I was in the middle of it all.

On Monday morning, September 24, 1984, I met a new patient, a forty-year-old former smoker who worked in politics and just had a heart attack.

CHAPTER THREE:

Before the Fall

I'm not afraid to die; I just don't want to be there when it happens."
—WOODY ALLEN

Mike Ranville:

For as long as I can remember I have been in love with the story. Thanks to a creative nun who fostered that interest, the story would dominate my professional and personal life, and, in the process, prove to be part of my downfall.

I grew up in a large family, six boys and two girls. In addition to being a door-to-door retail milkman, Dad was also a coach. With six boys roaming the house, we all fed on each other's love of athletics. A few years ago at a family gathering, not long after the last sibling had left home, Mom offered the astute observation, "This past week is the first I can ever remember where there wasn't a jock strap in the wash." Hard to believe a jock strap could play such a prominent role in family lore.

I played sports, football, and baseball in particular. At five feet eight inches I didn't even bother processing fantasies about basketball, although I usually made the team as the twelfth or thirteenth man, or more accurately, the final spot on the roster. As far as I was concerned, the only purpose basketball served was to keep the legs in shape between football and baseball season.

Although I did receive all-league honors in football and baseball, I was not a gifted athlete. Dad always said I was small but made up for it by being slow. Slow maybe, but I had endurance, demonstrated early in the two-a-day football practices, usually conducted in high humidity during the last week of August. A staple of those two-a-days was the dreaded mile run, in full pads. I usually finished early in the pack right along with the running backs. I loved that I could run forever.

I mention the mile run not to impress but to underscore that my one-time facility for endurance only compounded the frustration years later when a failing heart provoked a shortness of breath while walking from one room to another.

I always felt it a bit lofty to call myself a writer—David McCullough, Doris Kearns Goodwin, David Halberstam are writers—I just wrote an occasional speech or magazine article. Upon reflection, though, I spent most of my adult life making a living pounding a keyboard.

In high school I was on the school paper. Sister Marie Jude was as tough an editor as I would ever encounter, but she loved a good story, and, to my benefit, insisted it be told well. Life as a writer was too much of a pipe dream, but I never lost my love for hearing, telling and, maybe someday, even writing a good story.

In college I wrestled valiantly with tests, especially those tricky objective tests where there could be any number of right answers. Many a grade was saved, however, by turning in a well-researched, well-crafted paper that, thanks to Sister Marie Jude, usually included some sort of interesting and hopefully remembered story. While others pulled all-nighters before a test, I sought my grade weeks earlier while writing a paper, laboring over the right turn of phrase that parroted the professor's lectures, and included a valued anecdote to deploy at just the right juncture. While not a three-point student, I was more than happy with my gentleman's two-point five.

Having spent most of my professional life in the political arena, I learned early that control is everything, that information is power. And one of the most effective ways to control a project or group was volunteering to do the wretched first draft, a task studiously avoided by most. That first draft involved reducing to writing the purpose and goals of the group and laying out the next step in the process. It was much easier to offer criticism, but I discovered there first had to be something to criticize. And it was amazing how much of the content presented in that first draft survived. The burden of proof for altering that initial effort was on those who wanted something excised or changed.

I discovered a talent for writing speeches. In politics if you can make someone look good you have value. I didn't mind the anonymity. My reward arrived with the morning paper and an article that quoted the speech I wrote; even better if that article included one of my carefully honed phrases. Some who write speeches resent the applause directed at the speech-giver after delivering a speech they wrote. Not me; I remind myself of the directive Franklin Roosevelt delivered to his cadre of writers on the morning after his inauguration—"All staffers should have a passion for anonymity." He's right. If you want credit for a speech, run for office.

Whenever possible, the reports I wrote as a political staffer would contain some form of story to reinforce a point. If nothing else, I hoped the story would be remembered, and, more often than not, it was.

I started writing magazine articles under my own name. Not only did the money enhance the beer fund, but it also gave the ego an occasional boost.

Then I encountered a great story, one that many newspaper friends say they wait a lifetime for—the case of Milo Radulovich. Milo's page in history was assured when Edward R. Murrow and Fred Friendly drew on his case to inflict the first telling blow against Senator Joseph McCarthy in 1953. I wrote a book on the case, one of the readers was actor, writer, and producer George Clooney, who used my resurrected story for the first part of his acclaimed movie, *Good Night and Good Luck*. It was nominated for six academy awards, including best movie and actor.

I didn't appreciate it back then, but writing, although personally rewarding, was ruining my health, my heart in particular.

While I never took notice then, I learned many writers are heavy smokers. Recalling my hours at the keyboard, I now know why.

I would write a paragraph then light up a cigarette to review what I had just written. When there were enough paragraphs to fill a page, I lit up another cigarette to critique that page. Normally, mine was a pack-a-day-habit; that in and of itself a cardiac time bomb. While writing, especially during those glorious spurts when the adrenaline is flowing, I could easily consume an entire pack in a few hours. Concern for the hacking cough and occasional shortness of breath was subordinated to the joy and sense of accomplishment that accompanied the crafting of a graceful sentence.

The habit of smoking was easily acquired. The tobacco companies surely laughed derisively at me and other smokers whenever they reviewed their profit and loss statements.

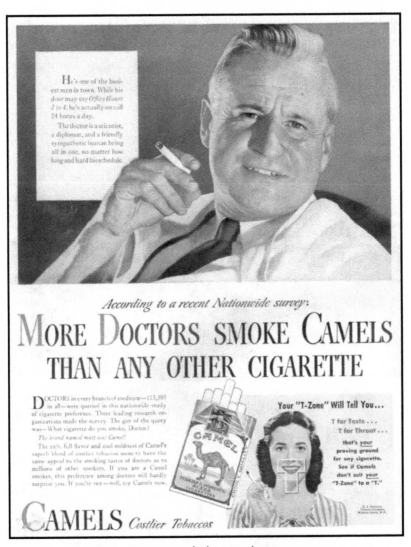

Everyone smoked – even doctors.

I started smoking in high school, nothing regular, just on those occasions when I desperately sought to project maturity and coolness. But why not? Everyone smoked; athletes, doctors, coaches, priests, my dad. Everyone who played an important role in my life (or so it seemed) smoked. Doctors and professional athletes even endorsed certain brands of cigarettes on the back of magazines. The heroes in movies cultivated lighting a cigarette into an art that caused women to swoon. The Marlboro commercials on television left the unmistakable impression that smoking translated into rugged manliness. How could the raging hormones of an insecure teen-ager reject all the testosterone a cigarette promised?

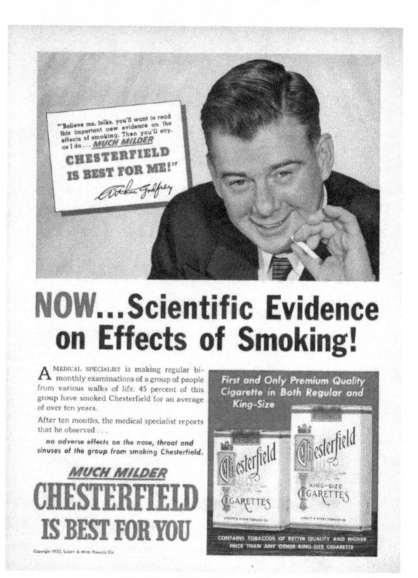

"No adverse effects" from smoking.

Further, government had yet to identify tobacco as a taxable source of revenue. Cigarettes were cheap. Stores rendered only a nodding glance to a law that required the purchaser of tobacco be eighteen years of age.

Fast food also invaded the nation when I was in high school. Only fifteen cents for a hamburger—I'll have three, and throw in some fries, too. No diet coke back then, we drank the real stuff.

More often than not entertainment consisted of a six-pack, riding around and singing oldies. We thought we were cool. Good friend Don Novak looked older and sported a continuous five o'clock shadow. He would turn his high school class ring around so it looked like a wedding band. We would meet at the checkout counter and I would feign surprise over running into "Uncle Don." While the cashier was tabulating the purchase, Don was busy with our carefully choreographed diversionary tactic—absent-mindedly reaching into his wallet to pay for the beer and asking me how the family was doing. While no academy awards were ever recorded, it was apparently convincing.

We drank the beer, ate potato chips, smoked incessantly, and then rounded out the night with a trip to McDonalds. And we did this far too many times. "Uncle Don" Novak died of heart problems at a young age.

At the age of twenty-two the Vietnam buildup was well underway and, after wrestling valiantly with my local draft board on the definition of a student deferment, I joined the United States Air Force. Cigarettes at the base commissary were dirt cheap. Even the lowest ranking enlisted man could afford to smoke. I realized years later the tobacco companies knew exactly what they were doing; establishing a smoking regimen early in life and reaping the benefits of that habit for a lifetime.

Mine was not the first generation who fell victim to the seductive strategy of big tobacco. My dad, who served with distinction in World War II, spoke of the magnanimous gesture tendered by the tobacco companies— free cigarettes. Nothing was too good for our boys in uniform. Big tobacco smugly waited patiently to realize the lifelong benefits of their patriotism, a GI hooked forever on their product. Cheap cigarettes were nothing more than an investment that would pay off handsomely someday.

Messages warning of the danger inherent in smoking were little more than a small and annoying voice that fell on deaf ears. The seductive commercials continued. Smoking was linked to fun.

The government was no help. Annually, congress approved valued subsidies for tobacco farmers. If cotton was king, tobacco surely was queen.

All this and much more was the package I had become as I wrote my reports, speeches, articles, and book. Each draft was evidenced by a crumpled cellophane wrapper that once held twenty cigarettes; and each pack of twenty cigarettes represented yet another carefully charted step in the journey to Ingham Medical Hospital on a Sunday night in the fall of 1984.

While cigarettes definitely were in the driver's seat on that trip to Ingham Medical, they had plenty of company. A positive byproduct of a life in politics is the gifted storytellers. Enjoying a few drinks after work while listening to grand and glorious tales of the world inhabited by elected officialdom, was a celebration of the story I so dearly loved. The tales were made all the better with a few drinks, and the drinks made better by high calorie, cholesterol-laden snacks. I had no concept of lifestyle. The heroes in my universe were those who could hold their drink and had great timing when delivering the punch line of a story. Sure, I'll have another beer, and bring another order of those chicken wings, too.

The Heart Attack

The third week in September 1984 was Indian summer at its very best in mid-Michigan. The temperatures were warm but not uncomfortable. The turning fall colors presented Mother Nature at her finest. September is the best time of year for us sports fans. Baseball is well into the drama of its annual pennant drives, and football is just beginning.

On Saturday, September 22, my nine-year-old daughter Mara, and I journeyed to old Tiger Stadium to watch Detroit do battle with the hated Yankees. Back then, baseball was still occasionally played during the day, as God intended. To my unending delight Mara demonstrated an interest in the grand ol' game, spurred on I'm sure by the fact that our Tigers took up residence in first place on opening day and remained there for the rest of the season.

Mara is an avid reader. Her insatiable curiosity that year was directed at baseball history. She read about baseball and quizzed me endlessly about games I watched with my Dad when I was her age. On the ride to the game that day I regaled her with tales of Frank Lary, a Tiger pitcher from my youth. He was also known as "Taters" and the "Yankee Killer," and always seemed to rise to the occasion when pitching against the Bronx Bombers.

It was a great dad 'n daughter day; the Tigers punctuating the perfect outing with a 6-0 win.

On the way home I wasn't nearly as expansive. For some reason my jaw hurt, and I didn't know why. Apart from a hot dog and popcorn, I hadn't eaten anything that would put a strain on my jaw. But the pain was more than just annoying, it was constant and had mushroomed into full-fledged discomfort.

The next morning the pain was gone and I was about to partake of the second phase of September's greatest offerings and watch the Lions and Vikings game at my brother's house. He lived less than a mile away; it was another gorgeous day so I rode my bike.

The only thing memorable about the game was how the Lions gave it away in the last minute. Sure-handed Robbie Martin dropped a punt that was recovered by Minnesota, enabling the Vikings to eke out a 29-28 win.

Pedaling my way home I noticed a slight pain in my chest. Like the jaw discomfort from the previous day; it wasn't debilitating, just uncomfortable and annoying. By ten o'clock that night, though, that pain was far more acute and convincing. It was steady, and showed no signs of subsiding.

Thoughts of my father came to mind. A heavy smoker, he suffered a heart attack at age thirty-eight, and then another at forty-five that he did not survive. Dad was a door-to-door milkman, working his route that day.

My mother was out shopping and thought she would surprise him and stop by to say hi. She found him slumped over in his truck. True or not, the doctor at the hospital graciously informed her that he died instantly. I was forty and wondered if "instantaneous death" was circling overhead.

After his first heart attack the doctor told Dad he should probably stop smoking. During a checkup a few months later Dad complained that not smoking made him nervous and edgy. Such was the state of cardiac care in 1958 that he was told by the doctor if it bothered him that much then he should resume smoking. Not surprisingly, as any smoker would have, he quickly resumed smoking.

Sitting on the edge of the bed that night, my chest heaving with a persistent pain, I sloughed off the notion that I was having a heart attack. After all, I had quit smoking the previous November. It had to be some form of indigestion.

I learned later that intuition is one of the most accurate indicators of a patient's condition. And this patient's intuition was telling him it was not mere indigestion. I told my wife Carol what was happening. She was quick and decisive; we were going into emergency. Normally I would have pushed back; not this time. I quickly agreed. She made arrangements to have someone come over and stay with Mara.

After the first of what would be many electrocardiograms in my life, I learned I was indeed having a heart attack.

I asked the nurse if there was a priest available. I took solace in the biblical story of the prodigal son, and the great rejoicing when a sinner returned to the flock. Shortly, our local priest arrived. Far from their intended comfort, the last rites are unnerving.

My first question to Dr. Bob Leeser, our family doctor and friend, was, "Am I going to die?" Not wanting to create any additional anxiety he patted my chest and said I was going to be fine. As a precaution, though, he transferred me to the Ingham Medical Facility, a thirty-minute ride to Lansing, where they could run more extensive tests. It was my first ambulance ride. Anxiety, however, did not subside when the driver turned on the flashing lights and drove much faster than I thought necessary. I quickly discerned this was far from routine.

An emergency room doctor was waiting for us at Ingham Medical. He immediately asked about the pain; how it felt, how long had I been experiencing it, when it started. After indicating I first noticed it while pedaling home after the Lions game, he made me laugh when he commented, "Must have started when Robbie Martin dropped that punt."

The next few hours are hazy. I drifted in and out of a restless sleep. I learned I was in the Intensive Care Unit and recall getting a sponge bath from a nurse who brought needed relief to a clammy feeling that had set in.

Carol called my office; obviously, I would not be going to work that day. Shortly thereafter my partner and close friend, Joe Garcia, appeared. I heard the nurse telling him that my condition was such that he could not see me. I worked in the political arena for a public relations/lobbying firm. In politics you learn to think on your feet, and that's exactly what Joe did. I chuckled again when I heard him tell the nurse that he was an attorney, which he was, and had been summoned by the family, which was pure fabrication. He was ushered in and told me not to worry, that he would ensure all appointments on my calendar would be kept. That was a relief.

Later that day I was transferred to a regular hospital room. While Carol was dozing in a chair, I took note of all the wires that were monitoring my every move and heartbeat, and wondered aloud, "What the hell am I doing here?"

I took stock.

I was only forty years old. Didn't smoke, or at least had quit months earlier—that should count for something. I prided myself on being able to handle the pressure that was a constant companion of my job. Okay, so I occasionally skipped lunch and grabbed whatever was handy in the office, more than likely M&M Peanuts or Nutter-Butter cookies, both of which were kept in plentiful supply for clients to munch on during meetings.

I was a moderate drinker, nothing excessive. But I did enjoy bringing the day to a proper close at happy hour. You don't just sip a beer or three at happy hour—appetizers all around.

My job required a lot of entertaining, much of which was accomplished during a meal. For me, large dinners at up-scale restaurants were part of the job. For my guests, a night of exquisite dining represented only an infrequent outing. And because I was buying, they would order an expensive, high-calorie meal with all the trimmings; drinks before, during, and after. And, more often than not, dessert. For them it was a time to splurge. My guests likely played an important role in the proceeds on my firm's profit and loss statement, so, not wanting them to feel out of place, I would order accordingly.

I finally acknowledged maybe all that entertaining had contributed to the suits feeling a little tighter. But I was active; still contributed to the softball team I played on with my buddies in the summer, water-skied at the lake with my daughter, nieces and nephews. I had no problem going up and down the stairs at home, and could still play a spirited game of wiffleball with the kids next door at the cottage.

Then reality hit. I'd just had a heart attack. While out of Intensive Care, I suspected all was not well when I was told not to leave the bed without assistance, which included using the rest room.

I really became concerned. Would I ever be a husband again? A father? Would I be able to provide for my family? Would I be a burden on them? How long was I going to live? Not easy questions, but lying on my back in a hospital, they consumed me. And I didn't have the answers.

Had only a few hours passed since I was thoroughly enjoying life at Tiger Stadium with my daughter? No one could ask for a more perfect day. And now I was attached to a sea of wires and couldn't even take a whiz without permission.

While anxiously tethered to a hospital bed, and with the incessant bleeping of machines as my only entertainment, my mind turned time and again to the confrontation with my own mortality.

Years earlier I read Faulkner's As I Lay Dying. At the time I thought it to be nothing more than a good story, rich in its representation of the Old South. Now, maudlin as it seemed, the plight of Addie Bundren as she awaited death, her family and life passing before her, took on a special meaning. The writer in me wanted to record the moment; the patient was scared as hell.

While he was by no means a priest, shortly thereafter, Dr. Michael James walked into my room, and my life. Things would never be quite the same again.

CHAPTER FOUR:

What Is A Heart Attack— And Why Did I Have One?

"To prevent a heart attack take one aspirin every day.
Take it out for a run; take it out to the gym, then take it for a bike ride..."
—RANDY GLASBERGEN

Dr. Michael James:

Mike Ranville had a heart attack on September 23, 1984. He just happened to be at the right place at the right time.

In 1966, his father died suddenly at age forty-five—from a heart attack. His father, Mike's grandfather, died suddenly of a stroke in 1946 at fifty-eight. Detect a pattern?

In the intervening years, great strides were realized in the body of research regarding treatment of heart patients. We still can't do anything regarding a more judicious selection of parents, but we can now claim heart disease is no longer a death sentence, or even a cessation of a productive life.

Mike was fortunate because I practice at the Thoracic Cardiovascular Institute (TCI). That's not a commercial for our practice; rather it underscores the importance of keeping pace with the most recent research

63

in the field of cardiology in general and treatment methods in particular. Along with many other practices, successful patient outcomes are closely linked with a dogged adherence to keeping abreast with the research.

In 1905, heart disease replaced tuberculosis and pneumonia as the leading killer in the United States. More than a century later it has yet to relinquish that dubious distinction. That single statement governed my decision to specialize in cardiology and drives me still today.

In the public arena there are many misconceptions regarding problems with the heart, especially when someone is called on to convey to others the condition of a family member or loved one. Armchair diagnoses frequently involve employing such statements as, "She had a massive heart attack," or "He has three blocked arteries and they don't know how, but he is still living." Ahh, the ubiquitous "they", invoked as a ready reference to assign credibility to any opinion, correct or not. As a member of the family of "they", I know that first impressions, inaccurate as they might be, are not quickly discarded and often lead to a lack of understanding of heart problems in general, and heart attacks in particular. If you want to know what they are saying, ask "them".

When it came to creating the human body, God must have vacillated between making it easy or making it difficult.

In the "making it easy" scenario, God created an amazing array of functional parts. But He made provisions for times when some of those parts couldn't perform. Two eyes are nice, but not crucial. Many successful athletes don't have ten toes or fingers. And you can actually survive on 10 percent of your liver. I have told several of my golf and ski buddies that I have an extra liver in the freezer in case they finish off their last 10%.

For those enjoying a cocktail while reading this, relax. The same is true for your heart. Although it functions best when all three arteries are working, there are many survivors doing well on two and sometimes one patent coronary artery. It was only in the past forty years that we finally started getting it right.

In 1969, during my residency at the Chicago College of Osteopathic Medicine, it was painfully evident that people dying of heart attacks were victims of arrhythmias that were preventable if caught early. However, they were still dying of cardiogenic shock, a condition where the heart suddenly can't pump enough blood to meet the body's needs. Sadly, that's one area where little progress had been realized.

There was enough data to support the notion that if patients were carefully monitored and nurses were trained to recognize fatal arrhythmias, and if those nurses were sanctioned to administer immediate treatment, many lives could be saved. But we were still treating the complications of a heart attack and not attacking the fundamental cause.

To those of us who were discouraged and sought an acceleration of the research, we took comfort in the fact that hospital mortality for heart attacks was now 15 percent, a marked improvement from the 30 percent of the 1950s before coronary care units (CCUs). We focused on pain management and suppression of arrhythmias.

We also embarked on a mission to educate the public, urging potential victims to seek medical assistance from a hospital as soon as possible after symptoms appeared in order to prevent fatal arrhythmias. Further, there was ample evidence to support the notion that if paramedics were authorized to administer preventive medications, even more lives could be saved. Specifically, once paramedics arrived on the scene they could now administer fifty milligrams of Lidocaine subcutaneously, a procedure designed to prevent arrhythmias.

The field of cardiac care was growing rapidly. It was now known as Invasive Cardiology and Coronary Bypass Surgery. Cardiac surgeons were "kings of the jungle." The bypass procedure, though, was only being performed on chronically diseased vessels and had no effect on the acutely occluded vessel. And we were again treating the diseased vessels, not preventing the development of plaque.

And plaque is critical.

Rare is the heart attack victim who has plaque-free arteries. By way of an understandable analogy, I tell patients that plaque is best illustrated by visualizing placement of an egg yolk on the windowsill. Initially it is soft and gooey. After a day or so it develops a crust. Eventually it becomes hard and crisp like chalk.

The plaque is a combination of cholesterol crystals and colloid. It accumulates over a period of time like silt at the bottom of a river bed.

Cholesterol was identified as a major culprit of heart attacks in a longitudinal study of the population of Framingham, Massachusetts, that began in 1948 and was revisited and refined a number of times. Variations of the study continue to this day.

According to the Framingham study, the average cholesterol level of heart attack victims in the United States was a lofty two hundred and forty-five. When the study was expanded to include other countries, we learned cholesterol levels in the United States were significantly higher. Notably, the heart attack ratio in Japan and Germany was miniscule when compared to that of America.

However, after World War II, when those countries became more westernized – read "adopted a Western diet"—their heart attack rates accelerated. Conversely, our rates dropped, a fact attributed to growing dietary discretion and use of cholesterol-lowering drugs, especially the statins. (Many share my firm belief that these are miracle drugs.) Also, while difficult to quantify, we began to realize the importance of daily exercise and the immediate benefits associated with a cessation of smoking.

What might seem logical—that plaque continues to accumulate, exact a burden, and then finally closes off the artery causing a heart attack—is not the case. Actually, the plaque ruptures and bleeds and we clot it. It is either the fibrous capsule that tears, or the center that explodes like a volcano creating a hemorrhage of mammoth proportions within the vessel. This is where luck enters the game.

In some instances, the patient dies suddenly. The plaque lodges at a strategic position within the arteries where it affects the electrical system and causes a fatal arrhythmia. More often than not, ventricular fibrillation occurs; the heart quivers prompting a termination of circulation and a precipitous drop in blood pressure or a complete heart block. There is a disconnect of electrical output from the top of the heart to the bottom.

Put simply, the top of the heart no longer beats in sync with the bottom. In order to save the patient from severe mental problems because of loss of oxygen to the brain, circulation needs to be restored within four minutes.

If the patient does not die suddenly, severe chest discomfort is experienced. While not a euphemism for severe chest pain, "discomfort" is the preferred term because the sensation is often described as "an elephant sitting on my chest," a feeling of impending doom and an aching in the left jaw. In older patients, severe shortness of breath is the second most common symptom.

In women the symptoms can be different: not as direct, but a sensation of just not feeling right and shortness of breath. Frequently, a heart attack in a woman is misdiagnosed.

As a general rule, the more severe the pain, the more heart muscle is lost. Not unlike the branches of a tree, if damage to a branch is in the portion closest to the tree, it affects the entire branch, and possibly the tree itself. Whatever contributes to the strength and health of that branch is weakened. Likewise, when all muscle that contributes to that tributary from the heart is destroyed, the vessel itself incurs damage; the more lost muscle, the more severe the symptoms.

We discovered from autopsies of soldiers that the formation of plaque can occur at a very early age. We learned young men in their twenties could have yellow streaks in their vessels, a gathering place for further accumulation of cholesterol crystals, adding to the existing plaque burden.

The source of plaque is neither surprising nor complex. Welcome to America. It is found primarily in our eating habits, in those delicious, high-saturated-fat diets. Compounding the problem is that plaque accumulation is aided and abetted by smoking cigarettes, a likely cause of damage to the artery. Those arteries, brimming with saturated fats, deposit further material onto the growing mound of plaque.

Diabetes, a frequent companion of heart attacks, increases the problem exponentially. When coupled with the inevitable aging process and hardening of the arteries, it all contributes to the perfect storm that culminates in an accumulated mass of plaque.

Enter the family genes. Coronary artery disease is strongly associated with family history. Some families, like Mike's, simply have a higher incidence of coronary artery disease than others. Genes notwithstanding, some of that family history might be proximity to smoking or poor diet, habits acquired in the home environment.

Finally, a sedentary lifestyle contributes greatly to the accumulation of the dreaded plaque.

The culprits are well known—high cholesterol, smoking, diabetes, age, family history, and lack of activity. Save for age and to a lesser extent family history, all are related to lifestyle decisions and in many ways controllable.

We were still plodding along, treating the complications of a heart attack. Defibrillation or ventricular fibrillation was common and very effective. Cardiogenic shock, when the patient loses at least 40 percent of the heart muscle, still carried an unacceptable 70 percent mortality rate.

Fast forward to 1984: in September, Mike Ranville entered my life. Mike worked as a lobbyist in the Michigan Capitol. He lived in Charlotte, a beautiful turn-of-the-century community located about fourteen miles from Lansing.

Mike was a ticking time bomb. He was a heavy smoker, at least a pack a day, sometimes more, for the previous twenty years. While he had quit smoking approximately a year earlier, like many newly minted non-smokers, he put on weight, in his case thirty pounds.

His professional life was constant pressure and consisted of several deadlines a day. He was "on-call" during the weekend, every weekend. The strain never abated. He was working an ongoing, stressful high wire act without benefit of a net. Balancing legislative egos with the demands of his clients was precarious enough, but in Mike's business there are no do-overs, no mulligans. It was success or failure, and he was painfully aware that failure does not have a second act.

Many nights were spent eating meals with those legislators and clients, the fellowship designed as a relaxed environment where the attempt was to bring both to agreement on an issue. And every one of those issues was "do or die." Small issues were for small people; insignificant players do not survive in a political environment. The meals were always full, characterized by rich foods, by mounds of saturated fat. Drinks before, during, and after. "And what'll you have for dessert, Senator?"

While he tried to exercise regularly, often there just wasn't the time, and after thirty extra pounds, there probably wasn't much inclination either.

His cardiac resume also included the renowned "sins of the father" risk factor, a family history of heart disease in general and a father who died suddenly at roughly the same age Mike was when he had his heart attack. The best advice I can give patients is to choose your parents prudently.

He was admitted to emergency on a Sunday night with that dreaded elephant sitting squarely on his chest. Initial treatment was provided by his very competent family physician, Dr. Robert Leeser. Dr. Leeser, who enjoys the deserved reputation of being an excellent diagnostician, quickly ascertained the resources of a larger, heart-oriented hospital were needed. Even though Mike had spent a good portion of the night at the community hospital, Dr. Leeser wisely ordered him transferred to Ingham Medical Center—and into my life.

Due to Mike's ongoing chest discomfort, which was still moderate to extreme, and his unusually high blood pressure of 160/140, and the fact that our institution could offer everything currently available in the realm of cardiac care, we willingly accepted the transfer request. From a personal standpoint, the reason I moved to Michigan was the opportunity to handle cases like Mike's. At Ingham Medical Center I had command of the most up-to-date equipment and procedures to draw on in caring for my patients.

There are three classic symptoms in the diagnosis of a heart attack.

1. Severe chest discomfort, which Mike certainly had. That elephant had definitely taken up residence on his chest.
2. Changes on the EKG. Every physician should be able to recognize those changes, especially those staffing emergency rooms.
3. Elevated enzymes. Enzymes are small particles that spill into the blood stream when there is tissue destruction or cell death. Mike's

enzymes were ten times the normal count, clearly indicating a major heart attack.

While he was not aware of it, Mike was about to benefit from the most current research in heart disease.

Mike was transferred because he was deemed an excellent candidate for thrombolysis, a procedure in which a patient is injected with a material called streptokinase, a derivative of the streptococcus bacteria, in order to break up blood clots. And we had to break up the clot that was clogging one or more of his coronary arteries to ensure a continuous flow of blood to the heart and brain.

The use of streptokinase was not a sure thing. Streptokinase is not specific to heart arteries. It also nullifies the body's ability to clot and is not easily reversible. The looming threat was that if the patient has any bleeding issues, even a fresh atrial or venous puncture, it could result in profuse bleeding.

He was sent to the Intensive Care Unit where his heart was constantly monitored. Fortunately, he had no significant arrhythmias and surprisingly no heart failure.

Our efforts focused on limiting the damage caused by an occluded artery. Recalling that heart arteries are like a tree with a trunk and multiple branches, the closer the occlusion to the trunk—the heart—the more heart muscle is in danger. Our efforts concentrated on opening the occluded artery.

We determined that the potential bleeding problem from the streptokinase was not worth the risk.

The slogan of the day was "Time is Muscle," a reference to the fact that the earlier the artery is opened the less damage will be incurred. From the time a patient enters the Emergency Room, staff is directed to get that patient to the catheterization lab and the occluded vessel opened as soon as possible. Currently, hospitals are being held to forty-five minutes or less—referred to as "Door to Balloon" time.

The resources of major hospitals are frequently not available in community hospitals. However, the community hospital can administer one or more of the clot-dissolving drugs that will enhance by 50 percent the chance of opening the damaged artery. Then the hospital must transfer the patient as quickly as possible to a cardiac center where an angioplasty— an emergency procedure to widen narrow or obstructed arteries or veins— can be conducted.

If I ever have a heart attack, my personal choice would be to do whatever is necessary to open that damaged artery as quickly as possible. If I am far removed from a cardiac center, then administer the thrombolytic—a drug to break up the clot—and move me out ASAP.

We were now about twelve hours from Mike's original occlusion and I concluded very little heart muscle could be saved. While Mike was treated with all the available tools, his artery was not opened within the desired time frame precluding the salvaging of some heart muscle.

While lucky in some respects, Mike was not in the right place at the right time.

After the first twenty-four hours following the heart attack he stabilized; most prominently, his chest discomfort was gone. His relief could be traced to the medications and the fact that he was already forming scar tissue in his heart. As with any scar there are no nerve fibers functioning, hence no pain. However, patients are carefully monitored for recurrent pain, which means there is still live tissue that is endangered by not getting enough fresh blood with oxygen to the heart muscle.

Bed rest was prescribed – but not absolute bed rest. Once stable, Mike was regularly roused from that bed to begin a routine of walking, a routine that must remain with him for the rest of his days. While trudging up and down the corridors of the hospital, he was still monitored and carefully watched for potentially fatal arrhythmias.

He was treated with long-acting nitroglycerin, geared to prevent further episodes of ischemia, an inadequate blood supply to the heart, and with a beta blocker, the cornerstone of cardiac care at the time. Beta-blockers remain the cornerstone of treatment for heart attacks to this day.

They decrease the amount of oxygen the heart needs to function without harming the efficiency of the heart. They also lower blood pressure, prevent arrhythmias, and lower the heart rate. More recently we have determined they help remodel the damaged heart, enabling it to work more efficiently. And not to be forgotten is aspirin, still a mainstay of treatment today because of its anti-clotting properties. Long acting nitrates have no mortality benefit and are no longer standard treatment post heart attack, they should only be used when patients have active angina—a pain in the chest due to an insufficient supply of blood to the heart—despite maximum medical therapy.

Throughout the thirty years since, Mike has remained on some form of beta blockers.

Mike the heart attack victim was far different than Mike the hospital patient. The heart attack victim was most compliant when it came to accepting significant changes in his diet and the need for regular exercise. However, when the hospital patient was told he needed to slow down, it was a directive not accepted gracefully. A revealing entry was included in the discharge notes dictated by the intern, "He had somewhat of a difficult time adjusting to the forced rest of the coronary care unit."

Here is where the art of medicine merges with science—and a little common sense.

The heart needs approximately six weeks to heal and form scar tissue at the area of the heart attack. For a patient like Mike—a stereotypical Type A personality—I needed as much information as possible to make the best decision before sending him home. Usually we would put the patient on a treadmill for a stress test, or administer a full catheterization[6]. In Mike's case we thought it best to do both.

Mike's catheterization was conducted approximately two weeks after his heart attack. I was hoping to find enough disease to recommend bypass surgery, but that was not the case. The results represented bad news and good news.

---

6   A catheterization is the most important diagnostic tool available to a cardiologist. It is
     examined closely in Chapter Five.

The bad news was that his heart had been severely compromised. His all-important ejection fraction—the amount of blood squeezed out with each heart beat—was 38 percent. Normal is 50 to 60 percent. To put it bluntly, the worse the ejection fraction, the worse the long-term prognosis.

The good news was that there were not enough blockages in any one artery to warrant a Coronary Artery Bypass Graft (CABG). Our alternative was medication. But this was more good news, because on average, the benefits of CABG surgery last ten years. After that, approximately half of the patients need another operation; the longer we can keep patients from procedures, generally the better off they are.

The parts issued by the good Lord for the initial version of the body are far better than any we can improvise. That not only includes the heart, but also knees, hips, and other advancements in modern medicine.

Mike was growing more frustrated by the day. Inactivity and relaxation were not staples in his wheelhouse. He pressed me hard for approval to return to work. My philosophy has always been to allow patients to return to a full lifestyle as soon as possible, and to paint as bright a picture as possible, as long as lives are not endangered. Sometimes it's not an easy call. A number of factors are taken under consideration; the ultimate decision being a combination of the subjective and the objective.

If the patient complains of ongoing chest discomfort, that could be ischemia, requiring immediate action with either coronary bypass surgery or with intracoronary artery stents. The other option is anti-anginal medication. Mike was on these prior to discharge, but we placed him on the treadmill just to be sure. Not only would a bout with the treadmill help monitor his symptoms of coronary artery disease but also assess his exercise tolerance and aerobic capacity, information that would determine what and how much activity would be safe for him. It would also enable us to see if we could induce chest discomfort or a nasty rhythm.

The results of the stress test are calculated in METS (Metabolic Equivalent over Time), a MET being a unit of exercise. For instance, it takes .5 METS to lie in bed all day and 14 METS to engage in any type of exercise the patient wants. The range for most people is between 7 and

8 METS; Mike did 12. I was as relieved as he was. He could return to work, both of us confident of his ability to handle the physical demands of his job.

Still to be determined, however, was how well he could accommodate the stress. In Mike's case it was a trade-off. I was convinced the stress he was encountering from not being able to work couldn't be any greater than that experienced while working. I told him he could go back to work.

One complication developed. Unfortunately, due to bronchial spasm, Mike was not able to tolerate the beta blocker of choice—a frequent side effect of beta blockers—limiting his medical options. The wheezing he developed was not dissimilar to the symptoms of asthma. I placed him on digitalis to get rid of the excess fluid.

While Mike was now out of the hospital, my training and commitment to cardiology proved to be beneficial to him. I was leading a dual professional life, as a teacher and a practicing cardiologist. Both my practice and my students were dependent on my staying current. Where the grinder once was only responsible for himself, he now directly and indirectly cradled the lives of others. A sobering thought, but I was far too busy to dwell on the enormity of the effect of my day-to-day decisions.

CHAPTER FIVE:

Catheterization— the Critical Tool

"There is no shortcut to achievement. Life requires thorough preparation. Veneer isn't worth anything."
—GEORGE WASHINGTON CARVER

Dr. Michael James:

One day while seeing patients in the clinic at Michigan State University, I received a call from the Dean of the Osteopathic School who said he needed a physical examination. While I thought it strange he was calling me, I obliged. Frankly, given his position, declining was not an option.

When I started taking his history it quickly became evident that his was a classic case of unstable angina. Whenever, for instance, he was in an airport walking from one terminal to another he would feel tightness in his chest. I looked him in the eye and told him he needed a catheterization.

"I know it," he said, "I just wanted to see if my new faculty was up to par." He had the catheterization the next day.

The results clearly indicated the Dean had left main coronary artery disease, "the widow-maker." It warranted emergency surgery. I told him he should stay in the hospital and surgery should be scheduled as soon as possible. He thanked me, said he would make his own decision, and walked out of the hospital straight for the Cleveland Clinic where he underwent triple bypass surgery.

The same scenario was repeated ten years later. He changed his lifestyle, took his medications as directed, and allowed me to treat him medically. He retired after many productive years as Dean, and lived well into his eighties. An outgrowth of my treating the Dean was that I became the chosen cardiologist for any faculty member who was experiencing a problem.

Why did I insist on a catheterization, and why did the Dean quickly agree? The catheterization history is as fascinating as its value.

A cardiac catheterization was first performed in 1929 by a German physician, Werner Forssman, who was only twenty-five years old at the time. Even though it was never tried on a live patient, he knew the method of entering the heart through a vessel in the arm was feasible. Forbidden to do the procedure on a live patient, he chose to do it on himself with a sterile, well-lubricated urethral catheter. He anesthetized his own left forearm and advanced the catheter sixty centimeters. He walked up two flights of stairs to the Radiology Department and, with a nurse holding a mirror, watched the catheter advance to the right atrium. While the catheter was not long enough to advance any further, he noted no untoward effects and no cardiac rhythm disturbance. Forssman's experiment advanced exponentially a critical understanding of the heart, prompting hemodynamic studies—the study of blood flow—to begin.

It would take twenty-eight years for the scientific community to recognize the noteworthy achievement. It wasn't until 1958 that someone dared enter the coronary arteries and produce an angiogram—a picture of the arteries that enabled identification of blockages. For their efforts Dr. Werner Forssman shared the 1956 Nobel Prize with Dr. Dickinson Richards of Columbia University.

In 1958, Dr. Mason Sones of the Cleveland Clinic accidentally engaged a twenty-six-year-old patient's right coronary artery and dye was mistakenly injected, without consequence. The result was the world's first coronary angiogram.

In November, 1976, things began to change for the cardiac surgeon and the interventional cardiologist. Andreas Gruentzig, a thirty-seven-year-old German-born physician, reported his research at the annual meeting of the American Heart Association that convened at the San Francisco Hilton Hotel. The prescient theme of the conference was "The Next Hundred Years."

At the time, the most effective method available to revascularize, or restore the flow of blood, to a clogged leg artery was to bypass the obstruction. Another approach, the Dotter Technique, used a series of increasingly larger catheters to widen the area of obstruction and improve blood flow away from the congested artery.

Gruentzig knew the Dotter Technique was not feasible for use in the coronary arteries because of their small diameter. However, he decided the obstructed artery could be "cracked open" with a small balloon. In fact, his paper to the American Medical Association (AMA) reported the results of animal studies and balloons. But there was no device yet available to accomplish that. In search of viable material and design, he worked with his wife and a few colleagues, primarily out of his kitchen, and developed a catheter with a resilient polyvinylchloride (PVC) balloon mounted on its tip. It was used to dilate the iliac artery in the leg.

His next step was to move into the coronary arteries. At that same gathering of the American Heart Association in 1976 he presented a paper on his findings. There were many doubters; some even scoffed at his findings, preliminary as they were. Undaunted, he issued an open call for assistance as he moved to the next stage of his research. There were no takers.

While no offers of help arose from the conference, his research intrigued Dr. Richard Myler of St. Mary's Hospital in San Francisco who offered the assistance of his hospital. Undaunted by the legion of skeptics, Gruentzig trudged onward.

Gruentzig and Myler would go on to earn their page in cardiac history when they performed the first coronary artery balloon angioplasty.

The prospects for complications were both many and serious, making the presence of a backup cardiac surgeon crucial:

- The balloon could rupture the artery and cause the pericardial sac to fill with blood and compress the heart with potentially fatal results.
- Plaque is not perfectly symmetrical and when the balloon inflates the plaque is cracked at its weakest point, which can lead to either a dissection that could split the vessel distally, or to small fragments that could break off and cause a heart attack.
- While the balloon is inflated the patient might not tolerate the vessel being obstructed, creating the potential for arrhythmia.
- The wire could break off or get stuck in the plaque and not be able to be pulled back.
- The balloon could rupture and get trapped in the vessel.

The cardiac surgeon who stepped forward was Dr. Elias Hanna. Gruentzig and Hanna worked on patients already scheduled for bypass surgery. It was here that the catheterization technique as we know it today was refined.

On September 16, 1977, Adolph Bachman, a thirty-eight-year-old Swiss insurance salesman with a high grade obstruction in his left anterior descending artery, wanted to avoid cardiac surgery. The procedure was performed. All precautions were in place. The operating room was fully prepared to move quickly in the event of an emergency. An anesthesiologist and a surgeon were also present.

The patient was awake and after the first balloon inflation there were no EKG changes. A second inflation was done. The procedure was a resounding success and the discipline of Interventional Cardiology was born.

Significantly, in 1977, only a year after his research was met with skepticism at the American Heart Association, Gruentzig presented again at their annual conference, this time on his first four angioplasty cases. He received a standing ovation.

Gruentzig became a celebrity and soon was recruited to Grady Memorial Hospital in Atlanta, Georgia, where he worked closely with Dr. Spencer King III of Emory University, among others. Up until his untimely death on October 27, 1985, Gruentzig was providing multiple courses in Percutaneous Coronary Intervention (PTCA).

On October 27, 1985, while he was at the controls, Andreas Gruentzig and his wife died in a plane crash over Georgia. The father of Interventional Cardiology was only forty-six at the time of his death.

***

From day one I loved the cath lab. It is exciting, definitive, and rife with pressure. While information yielded by a catheterization is critical to an accurate diagnosis and subsequent treatment program, the procedure is not without risk. It requires a steady, knowledgeable, confident, and able hand at the till.

One mistake can result in a stroke, an aortic dissection, or a coronary dissection, all of which could lead to death. There is also the danger of minor complications that can easily mushroom, such as a large hematoma, a swelling caused by a break in the wall of a blood vessel, triggered by a misdirected stick in the femoral artery. A hematoma can linger for months and often requires surgery to correct the problem.

I always admired the great athletes who not only want the ball but demand it when the game is on the line. Like the great athletes, in the cath lab many doctors—me included—demand the ball. This is not a confidence borne of ego or arrogance, rather of experience and ability. Simply put, doctors are held responsible for their actions. As such, they must have control of the process. If I'm a patient on the catheterization table I want a doctor who demands the ball.

To illustrate, the cath lab team is similar to the crew of a jumbo jet. The doctor is the pilot, responsible for the activities of all on board—in this case the crew and especially the "passengers", the patients.

My cardiac crew consists of:

- A cardiovascular technician, the "co-pilot", qualified to assist in both the routine and the unforeseen, who intuitively has available the proper equipment necessary for the pilot to effectively carry out the procedure;
- A technician in the control panel charged with monitoring the intra-arterial pressures and continuous rhythm of the heart;
- An x-ray technician responsible for the million-dollar x-ray machine that records the necessary visual images of the heart's arteries and chambers;
- A rotating nurse responsible for monitoring the patient and administering the proper medications.

The old political axiom—"You can delegate authority but not responsibility" is alive and well in the cath lab.

The team is well trained and highly professional. A catheterization is a demanding procedure. Due to its utility, it is in high demand. It is not uncommon for the team to do as many as thirty to forty in a single day. Maintaining discipline and focus is critical. The doctor in charge must not relinquish control. Control in this case is not a reflection of ego, but of fulfilling the responsibility invested in directing the procedure. Going in, I make sure the team understands that all decisions are mine or go through me, as I am responsible for their mistakes as well as mine.

Given the import and delicate nature of a catheterization, the ability to hyper-concentrate in the cath lab is essential. Possessing the facility to instinctively discard the extraneous and focus in laser-like fashion on the situation at hand, especially during an emergency, is vital. Despite a sometimes deserved reputation for frenetic behavior during the conduct of my normal day, life slows for me during an emergency and I proceed, one carefully calculated step at a time. The triggered hyper-concentration has served me well.

Once during the middle of an angioplasty when the vessel was wired and the balloon was ready to be inflated, John Enders, one of the nurses in the control room frantically announced, "Kirsten (one of the Cardiac Care Unit nurses) just collapsed in the hall. We need help!"

I made sure my angioplasty patient was not in any danger, broke scrub, pulled the balloon back, tore off my lead, and charged into the hall. Kirsten was definitely down. All those around her, including the head CCU nurse, were panicked. But no one was helping Kirsten. She needed immediate assistance—from someone able to take charge and dissipate the growing pandemonium, to address her obvious medical needs. Kirsten's life, not spared feelings, was my chief concern.

I took sorely needed control, firmly ordered the head CCU nurse to "Calm down and pay attention. Get the gown off." Gown removed, everything went noticeably silent; all were waiting for the next order.

Intuitively I knew what needed to be done, and didn't hesitate. The orders were clear, quick and definite – "John, get a pair of scissors and expose her chest. Get the paddles and 'buzz her' (defibrillate)." One shock was all it took and her rhythm was restored. I learned later that my abruptness had offended some on the makeshift team that had saved Kirsten's life. I went back to the cath lab and finished the angioplasty, without incident.

When all was done, and I could finally reflect on the angioplasty and Kirsten's simultaneous arresting in the hall, the realization hit me; in only an instant I had saved two lives. Summoning the pilot and jumbo jet analogy once more, it was a successful emergency landing that might never occur again. But a pilot took charge and a disaster was avoided.

It was a rare personal moment. After years of preparation, of waging war with standardized tests, of competing with the silver spoons of the world, "the grinder" was now a healer. It is the highest of accolades and I am not about to relinquish that vigorously pursued and coveted credential.

While certainly not unique to me, the ability to swat aside the superfluous and immediately beckon years of training, and do so for the most noble of reasons, characterizes the poise and assurance of those who demand the ball. Like the gifted athlete, they make that demand because they can produce—and in the cath lab, they save lives.

My playing field is not a huge stadium; it is a hospital, a cath lab, and countless other medical venues. Adoring fans do not gather outside the cath lab screaming, "Miiiikeee! Miiiikeee!" And the consequences of how well I perform far exceed in importance the prestige of a won-loss column in the morning paper.

Someday I might be the guy who arrests in the hall. If so, I want the person in charge to be totally in control, confident of what to do next. And I sure don't want someone who is concerned that the severity of tone in the voice might bruise some feelings. On the contrary, I want a trained medical professional directing activities; one who can quickly assess the problem, instinctively decide what needs to be done, and can communicate orders in a firm and convincing fashion—no shades of gray. If the directives lack tact, and are interpreted as rude or arrogant, so be it. I want the tactless cardiologist who demands the ball.

***

The most important tool available to the interventional cardiologist is the catheterization lab, where the definitive diagnosis is made. My years in and around the lab bring to mind certain catch phrases that help illustrate what happens there, and why it is important.

"Non-invasive equals non-diagnostic...The Dye don't lie...Echo Schmeko, Nuke Puke, Cath yea." (Sorry—Insider catheterization baseball...)

Catheterization is an invasive procedure. Without it, though, the diagnosis is severely lacking. Why settle for another procedure with a 70 percent accuracy rate when 100 percent is available in the cath lab?

When I finished my Fellowship in 1974, all we were doing in the cath lab was providing diagnoses. If a mechanical correction of the problem was warranted, the cardiac surgeon was brought in and the patient sent to the operating room. The cardiologist made the diagnosis, the surgeon fixed it. Now in 2018, the volume of cardiac surgery as well as the income of cardiac surgeons is down because of stents. This is sad because most cardiac surgeons are in their mid-fifties and will soon be retiring. There was a time in the not too distant past when there were four hundred applicants for fifty vacancies—last year only fifty of those spots were filled and who knows how qualified the applicants were? In the future, community hospitals may abandon cardiac surgery altogether and a vital medical procedure might be performed only in large hospitals or in academic centers.

Early in my career at the University of Michigan I was enamored with the vast amounts of critical information cardiac catheterization yielded, and wanted to be as proficient as possible with this procedure. At the time, catheterizations were only performed by going through the arm with a cut down to the brachial artery. At nearby St. Joseph Hospital the procedure was being accomplished by entering the femoral artery in the groin.

The arm approach was known as the Sones technique, named after Dr. Mason Sones from the Cleveland Clinic. The problem with the arm approach was that a cardiologist not trained in vascular surgery was opening a brachial artery and maneuvering a catheter through that artery, around the shoulder, and down to the origin of the coronary arteries—and in the process, injecting contrast to outline the lumens, or cross sectional diameter of a tube, to identify high grade plaques in those vessels. The arm approach also required a number of people because the artery had to be stitched back together. Additionally, it compromised circulation. Finally, because this was a teaching hospital, there were many who had to learn this important process. Some Fellows had good technique, and to be blunt, some did not. Who suffered as a result of the "did-nots"? The patients did.

Not far away at St. Joe's, the private hospital, they were doing catheterizations via the Judkins technique that utilized the groin as a point of entry as opposed to the arm. Named after Dr. Melvin Paul Judkins, the groin approach engaged the femoral artery with a needle stick. It placed a sheath in the vessel and then used three preformed catheters to address the coronary arteries. It secured the same pictures without having to surgically repair the artery. Simply holding pressure for ten minutes usually stopped the bleeding. This seemed a much simpler procedure to acquire the same information, so I spent as much time as possible at St. Joseph's mastering the technique.

While little was made of it publicly—and understandably so—when legendary Michigan football coach Bo Schembechler needed bypass surgery and cardiac care, it was all done at St. Joe's rather than the university hospital—surely a severe blow to the prestige of the surgical team at the University of Michigan.

At this point I was in my second year. After I learned the Judkins technique, I approached the staff at the University of Michigan and asked why they continued to embrace the outdated Sones method, when only two miles away the procedure was accomplished in half the time, yielded the same data, and was conducted with far fewer complications. The answer was, "This is the way we've always done it, and those guys are going to get in trouble if they continue their errant ways." It made no sense to me. But the day came when no matter how hard the University people tried, no matter how many catheters were deployed, they still could not engage the coronary arteries.

I enjoyed a reputation of having good hands, as they are called, asking if I could do what the guys at St. Joe's were doing. Life does not present many moments when you can truly "strut yer stuff." This ol' grinder sensed such a moment was before him. I moved quickly to borrow catheters from St. Joe's. In front of the entire catheterization team I secured all the data, without complication, and in a very short period of time. Shortly thereafter, the university hospital ordered the necessary equipment and changed from the Sones Technique to the Judkins Technique. For the record, I have never been a gloater. Despite great temptation, the ol' grinder wisely chose to take his victory lap in silence.

CHAPTER SIX:

"Marcus Welby, Where Are You When We Need You?"

"Never go to a doctor whose office plants have died."
—ERMA BOMBECK

Dr. Michael James:

On a Monday morning in the fall of 1984, I acquired a new patient. Over the weekend, Mike, a forty-year-old man with a family history of heart problems, a former smoker, and fast-food aficionado who worked in a high pressure field, had a heart attack. Talk about an apostle of the obvious.

That, in and of itself, is significant because given the nature and severity of his heart attack, statistically speaking, I should have attended his funeral years ago. His refusal to take up residence in that statistical category can, at least in part, be traced to the fact that he openly embraced a new life-style regimen that called for careful monitoring of diet and regular exercise. Moreover, he kept an eager and open mind to the rapid advancements in cardiac care during the past thirty years. He not only survived but thrived, and ably fulfilled his role as a husband and father to his family.

Not to minimize the lifestyle changes, but there is one other key factor that figured prominently in his survival – a close working relationship between Mike's family physician, Dr. Robert Leeser, and me.

Sadly, that critical relationship no longer holds the prominence it once did.

For as long as I can remember, the family physician was in charge of the patient. For some inexplicable reason, that notion has been abandoned. I clearly remember my student days from 1965 to 1969 when a specialist would not dare fashion a care program for a patient without first conferring with the family doctor; and God forbid if anything was done for a patient without knowledge of that family doctor.

Back then, though, family doctors actually visited patients in the hospital, wrote orders, and made the medical decisions regarding their care. They knew that patient well, knew the spouse, the children, even the family dog. When tough calls had to be made, especially an end-of-life decision, it was the family doctor who convened the discussion. More often than not that doctor was already aware of the patient's desire regarding what is now euphemistically known as "calling in the palliative care team."

I did a rotation in Waterville, Maine, between my sophomore and junior years and got to know "Hurry-up Harry," the prototype family doc. Harry could do it all, right in the office, when it came to basic medicine; tonsillectomies, baby deliveries, removal of small lesions. Moreover, if there was a patient admitted to the hospital via Emergency, he would find time to stop by during lunch for a visit. I recall a small boy who came to us with a pea stuck in his ear. Harry could not locate an appropriate instrument to remove it so he took a paper clip, bent it, and successfully pulled the pea out.

I came to appreciate and greatly admire those family doctors. Harry and his dedicated and knowledgeable cohorts were intimately involved in the care of their patients, and, make no mistake, those patients belonged to them; they hovered over them like a panther over her cubs.

The role of the family doctors, the all-knowing, pervasive care givers, persisted throughout my training. When I first arrived in Lansing, Michigan, I witnessed again the deference accorded the family doctors.

A typical day began at seven o'clock in the morning when all the physicians, specialists, and family doctors would gather in the doctors' cafeteria, just off from the main cafeteria. The television would be blaring and the conversation sometimes drifted to the stock market or a prominent sport story. The main thrust, however, was the patients under the care of these physicians. Soon the general surgeons were off to their operating rooms. This was the '70's, a time when internists were the "lords of the jungle" and would remain in the hospital most of the day to attend to the sicker patients. Relatively speaking there were not many sub-specialists, cardiology, pulmonary, and so on.

Later, after a day in the office, the family doctors would return to visit their hospitalized patients. They certainly knew more about our sub-specialties than we knew about their all-encompassing practice of medicine.

The family doctors were the products of broad training that exposed them not only to internal medicine but to the sub-specialties as well. I held those family doctors in the highest regard, and the years have done nothing to diminish that admiration. I admire their capacity to know the various diseases, the ability to make the final diagnosis—and that they are correct most of the time.

Conversely, I wanted to master one organ which, at least in my view, reduced the opportunity for error and enabled me to provide the best possible care for my patients. However, I actively sought the counsel of the family doctor, the patient being the beneficiary of our joint effort.

As time went on, save for a few who still need to be intricately involved in all aspects of patient care, the family doctors have all but disappeared from the hospital. With their departure they took a quality of hospital care that cannot be duplicated.

Some of my colleagues (frankly, the more haughty ones) view involvement from family physicians as meddlesome and counter-productive. Quite the opposite, they should welcome them with open arms. The family doctors know their patient and are trusted by the family. They can discern when a patient needs a hug, or a symbolic kick in the butt. That knowledge and trust can be especially helpful when a family is confronted with an end-of-life decision.

There are times when a patient's issues and deportment warrant tough love. The family physician is the appropriate individual to make that call, not some sensitivity major. It's a decision that should be rendered by a qualified medical person who knows the patient and the family, not a social worker from the Human Relations Department.

During one of his office visits, Mike and I got into a discussion of the important role played by his family doctor, Dr. Bob Leeser. He told me many stories that only reinforced my conviction that a family doctor plays an integral role in the lives of his patients.

When Mike's infant daughter was treated for dehydration, Dr. Leeser called their home a number of times during the next few days, "just to check on the little one." Who else but the family doctor can best ease the parent's' anxiety over a sick baby? When the head of the county commission needed to appoint someone to the tri-county mental health board[7], he consulted Dr. Leeser. Who else but the family doctor had a finger on the pulse of the community as he did? Mike also encountered a young couple who at one time were having some marital difficulties. They didn't want to talk to a therapist; they wanted to talk with Dr. Leeser, their family doctor, someone who enjoyed their unfailing trust.

When Mike got angry at work one day and broke his hand after slugging a file cabinet, it was Dr. Leeser who scolded him, telling him in no uncertain terms that his immaturity could have endangered his job, his ability to provide for his family. After learning what happened, Dr. Leeser's opening volley set the tone.

---

7   He recommended a respected local social worker, Carol Ranville, (Mike's wife) who
     supervised Protective Services for the county Department of Social Services and enjoyed a
     reputation for strong advocacy on behalf of the victims who came under her jurisdiction.
     She served on the Community Mental Health Board with distinction for a number of years.

"That's real smart," he lectured the would-be pugilist. Who else but the family doctor could mend a broken hand and provide unvarnished wisdom, and do so all in one visit?

As to my professional and personal relationship with Bob Leeser, he is absolutely one of the best family physicians I have ever encountered. My phone calls to him are promptly returned; likewise, I quickly get back to him. Those strong and frequently used channels of communication are directly responsible for Mike beating that statistical category.

Unfortunately, family physicians no longer regularly frequent the hospital. They stay in their offices and see a different patient every twelve minutes, carefully documenting the level of care so they can pay the four to six Full-Time Equivalents (FTE's) necessary to support each physician's practice.

The system has altered the practice of medicine. There are fewer and fewer Doctors in private practice, and that has changed the dynamics considerably. Their income depends on RVU's Relative Value Units (a unit of reimbursement for patient visits or procedures) and these are what the bean-counters use to evaluate the Doctor's value. It is simply not cost effective to do rounds once or twice daily and probably not very efficient. Enter the Hospitalist: basically a person that has completed a three year Internal Medicine residency and is responsible for taking care of any and all patients "admitted" to the hospital. Although well trained, they cannot possibly have the personal relationship that the family doctor established over many years.

And that's a shame.

After age sixty, the number of problems in the human body increase. It's a time when lumps appear, prostates enlarge, hearts begin to fail, and a time when that family doctor's steadying influence and comprehensive medical background is needed most. The probability for getting prostate cancer, for instance, increases with each passing year; at age seventy the chances are 70 percent.

The same doctor who for years treated the family's bronchitis, set their broken bones, delivered their babies, is now slowly giving way to medical care provided by a set of strangers. Not only is the invaluable intimate doctor-patient--family relationship a casualty, but the toll exacted on finite health care dollars is both significant and totally unnecessary. Who are these strangers who go by perplexing, unfamiliar names – hospitalist, intensivist, the palliative care team? If it wasn't so frustrating, it would be humorous.

I remember a patient telling me what it was like lying in bed, waiting for the seven minutes carefully allocated him during "rounds." He likened it to the Head Rat coming into the room, devotedly followed by three to five obedient blind mice. The Head Rat (the hospitalist) would bark orders or ask questions. Sometimes the questions were directed at the patient, other times at the three blind mice. Some of the queries were germane to the patient; others were intended to make a point with the resident, fellow, physician's assistant, or the nurse—the three blind mice. Depending on what day it was, there was a distinct possibility the three blind mice had never seen the patient before.

Later, another Head Rat arrives with an additional set of mice in tow. If the patient has a number of issues, up to twenty medical people could see him in one morning, when rounds are normally conducted. There is no time to get to know a patient, become familiar with a patient's family, to explain in some depth what may or may not happen with a pending procedure, to even know if a patient wants to live or die.

Is there ever time to sit down and discuss the entire case? Absolutely not! That's the job of the family doctor who is supposed to take over after discharge. At least that's what is called for in the grand design. In reality, the hospitalist assumes the family doctor will accept responsibility for the patient's care, and, barring information to the contrary, the family doctor assumes the hospitalist has completed the care.

Sorely-needed communication is little more than a rumor. There was a time when the family doctor and the specialist talked about that patient and jointly devised a carefully tailored program of care. But those meaningful conversations once held in the physicians' cafeteria at seven o'clock each morning, conversations that were critical to the recovery of the patient, no longer take place. The primary communication tool today is the discharge summary, often a hastily crafted document that may or may not accurately reflect what transgressed in the hospital.

For the patients who are really sick and end up in the Intensive Care Unit, they will be introduced to the intensivist. The intensivist is charged with shepherding the patient through the crisis. They will become familiar with the patient's blood pressure, lab work, chest x-rays, but have no idea who that patient actually is; not the family, not the job, not the patient's fears, nothing.

Recently, a good friend of mine, also a physician, was discharged from Intensive Care with a urinary catheter still in him. When his wife, a registered nurse, asked how often the catheter needed to be clamped, the ICU nurse curtly responded, "We just saved his life – he's out of here. Ask the nurses on the floor what to do. Good-bye!"

The current state of hospital care is heavily influenced by a mountain of rules and regulations, all geared toward achieving economies of scale. The hospitalist is under pressure to make sure the length of stay doesn't deviate from the criteria devised for the specific diagnosis. Every diagnosis includes a carefully delineated length of stay. Departing from that plan is highly frowned on. For the hospitalist and the intensivist, too many departures from that plan will warrant an explanation.

An additional vital sign has been added to the classics of blood pressure, pulse, and temperature: pain. Of course pain management is important, but a certain segment of the population (drug seekers, pain prescription addicts) have figured out that giving a poor grade regarding their treatment on the patient discharge satisfaction form, which can count against the doctor both for reimbursement and continuation of privileges, can get them better and more drugs. Some ER doctors are feeling forced to continue "managing" these patients' pain and let the government determine how to deal with these individuals.

The goal is to get the patient out as soon as possible into the hands of the family doctor, the same family doctor who is seeing a patient every twelve minutes. That family doctor will now receive a patient fresh out of the hospital who has four different diagnoses and whose prescriptions have been significantly altered. Moreover, the family doctor is charged with plowing through twenty to thirty pages of drivel from which must be extrapolated a treatment plan.

I don't see it getting better. If ever admitted to a hospital, I would give serious consideration to hiring a private nurse whose function would be to make sure that everyone who comes to see me carefully explains, in layman's terms, what is going to happen. Further, the purpose and dosage of every medication would be checked and re-checked.

We used to have the gate keeper, the family doctor. There are still excellent family doctors but their roll has changed dramatically. Although the hospitalist, the intensivist, and the specialists are all well trained they cannot possibly have the same relationship with the patient. This is especially important when it, comes time to decide to 'keep going" or to "know when to fold it, and to walk away'; to stop adding years to the life, and allow the patient to die with dignity.

I know I am old school and when I see what is happening in the world, I yearn for the "old days." This however is the age of specialization.

I look at major league baseball. There was a time when the starting pitcher pitched nine innings; maybe a reliever was needed if he tired. There was no pitch count, no long reliever, no switching to a left-handed or right-handed batter to accommodate "the odds," no ninth inning only closer. In football there was no platooning; if you played offense then you also played defense. There was no third down back, no long snapper, and no punt team. Is it better? Well I guess the product is better, but is it really better?

In medicine the training of the hospitalist, the intensivist, and the palliative care team is more extensive but is it better? I personally look at medicine and conclude there are about a thousand things that can go wrong and we can fix about 100. The rest is managing symptoms.

In cardiology we are not curing atherosclerosis we are replacing parts. In orthopedic surgery we are not curing arthritis and degenerative bone disease, we are replacing worn out parts. In surgery we are not curing diseased organs, we are removing them.

So it is here that the family doctor needs to be intimately involved in decisions. I have several colleagues who strictly adhere to that notion. I challenge the new generation to be as involved with their patients as their older peers are today. Do not abdicate your responsibility to your patients and relinquish critical decisions entirely to the "others."

Marcus Welby, where are you when we need you?

CHAPTER SEVEN:

"It's Okay to Sweat Again"

"I got underwear older than her."
—**Jud Heathcote**

Mike Ranville:

Following the heart attack I remained in the hospital for two wretched weeks.

At first it was all a novelty. I was suddenly, at least in my distorted view, the center of the universe. Friends called or stopped by – far too close for comfort to the ritual *paying our respects*. When Carol, visited she always had a list of people who "just wanted Mike to know I was thinking of him." I hail from a family of eight children. In addition to Mom, my brothers and sisters also kept in touch. People I hadn't heard from in years somehow learned of my heart attack and were added to Carol's daily list of well-wishers.

My nine-year-old daughter, Mara, was deemed too young to visit. The rules were bent, or maybe ignored, and seeing her walk into my hospital room was a great boost for morale. Just the presence of Carol and Mara was more important to my recovery than the latest advancement in cardiac care.

It was a storybook year for the Detroit Tigers. They began the season in grand fashion – nine straight wins, thirty-five out of the first forty – and never looked back. Interest throughout Michigan bordered on a feeding frenzy.

Tiger broadcaster George Kell and I were friends. We regularly had dinner when he came to Lansing to shoot television commercials for Capitol Savings and Loan. Near the end of the season, when the Tigers were in New York playing the Yankees, George took a moment to "wish my old buddy Mike Ranville the best after a recent health setback. Get off the DL (disabled list), Mike. We're gonna need you for the playoffs." A friend taped the game and I still have it, the George Kell greeting intact.

The cards, the calls, the flowers, numerous baseball books to fill the time during convalescence, the special message during a Tiger game— from storied Yankee stadium no less – it was heady stuff. The remembered visits, though, were from those who had suffered their own heart attacks and lived to tell about it. They significantly reduced my rapidly growing anxiety level.

Larry Tokarski, Michigan Governor James Blanchard's liaison to the legislature—a victim of two heart attacks—took time from his hectic schedule to visit. He had a calming effect.

"I know you're wondering if you'll ever be a father again, a husband, wondering if you'll be able to support your family," he said. "The answer is, yes, you will."

Coming from Larry, who not only was gainfully employed but held one of the most pressure-laden jobs in the Capitol, did wonders for my slowly deteriorating attitude. When a fruit basket arrived from the Governor, I knew Larry was responsible, but it was still a thoughtful gesture, very much appreciated. And I figured even if the Governor didn't actually send it, he at least had to know about it.

Gordy Gotts, president of the Michigan State Police Troopers Association—also a heart attack victim—reinforced what Larry said about life after the dreaded myocardial infarction. Gordy and I had logged many hours together building a successful legislative program for the Troopers

Association. In the process we became close friends. We knew each other too well for him to offer shallow, gratuitous comments. When he assured me everything would be fine and we would soon be roaming the Capitol together again, he wasn't trying to make me feel better. Like Larry, Gordy spoke from experience. It meant something.

My best friend, Bob Joseph, also communicated on a daily basis. Bob, an attorney who lives in the Washington, D.C. area, was prepared to book an immediate flight to Lansing "to do whatever needs to be done" – help with any legal problems, sort through the growing pile of paperwork my hospital stay was generating, stay with Mara while Carol spent time at the hospital (at Mara's insistence we never used the term "baby-sit"). And just be there in case I wanted to talk.

Now, after ten days, I was slated for discharge. While the thought of going home was nothing short of exhilarating, it paled, at least temporarily, to the knowledge that certain staples of a hospital stay were soon to be consigned to the rear view mirror.

I was leaving behind the mass of forever tangled wires attached to machines and monitors that recorded my every heartbeat. They were my constant and cumbersome companion on the many journeys up and down the corridors of the hospital. When sharing experiences with other heart patients, there is universal agreement that liberation from the wires contributes immeasurably to personal comfort.

I was abandoning the call button that robbed me of dignity and summoned a nurse to supervise even the most menial of tasks – such as using the bathroom.

I was bidding farewell to the technicians who drew blood from my scarred arms at all hours of the day and night. The irony of being constantly told "you need to rest" by constant interruptions to that rest was not lost on me.

How would I ever sleep again without the discomforting sounds of a hospital? Could daytime television survive without me?

Discharge from a hospital can be a trying procedure.

I recall being told I was going home; my spirits soared. But then I learned the entire medical community in the western hemisphere has to sign off before the volunteer actually wheels you down to the lobby.

Further, much of the paperwork fell to the already overworked nursing staff. They had other patients besides me demanding their time, and for some inexplicable reason it didn't seem to matter to them that my name was recently mentioned on a Tiger telecast.

So I sat and waited. And like that watched pot, waiting did not make the moment of discharge appear any quicker. Perhaps the system is carefully designed to render the patient all the more appreciative once the discharge becomes reality. Eventually, though, the moment arrived.

The ride home, even though routine, was eventful. The sights, sounds, and smells were appreciated as if being experienced for the first time. I recall stopping at a corner, waiting for the light to turn, and encountering the unmistakable fragrance of popcorn. I love popcorn.

Now that diet is critical I noticed how many fast-food establishments dotted the landscape. I remembered a comment from a dentist-friend who noticed a young child drinking a sugar-laden bottle of regular soda pop. "That kid doesn't know it," he said only half kiddingly, "but he's sending my kid to college." I thought to myself that fast-food establishments are doing the same for Dr. James.

Finally, home. What a treat to walk in the back door, stroll through the friendly confines of the kitchen and dining room, and then to the living room and my big easy chair. So much had happened since I left but so little had changed. Now I was safe, back in familiar and comfortable surroundings. Even the book I was reading the night of my heart attack sat undisturbed on the table next to the easy chair. So vivid is my recall of that moment I can say for certain that *Ironweed* by William Kennedy waited patiently for my return.

We live on a corner that has a high rate of pedestrian traffic. I wondered why so many people were out strolling; didn't they have somewhere to go? Why did they seem so calm? Absent was the urgency and intensity of the marketplace where until recently I held forth. Save for Saturdays and

Sundays, and an occasional holiday, I had never been home during the day. Daytime people are different. Life is slower, less deliberate.

Now, difficult as it was to accept, I was one of those daytime people. Where once the clock radio was cursed as the morning news dragged me from sleep, now it only served to tell time. I got up when I didn't want to sleep anymore. It was a drastic change not easily embraced by someone who always had someplace to go, something to do. All too soon, though, boredom and depression found their way to that easy chair.

Logically, I understood I was convalescing. Emotionally, I craved the adrenaline that heretofore coursed through my workday. What were my partners doing, right now, at this very moment? Were the needs of the clients I dealt with, the clients I had carefully nurtured throughout the years, being accorded the same quality of service I tried to provide? While I wanted to believe no one could do it as well as I did, the truth is I was not indispensable and the firm continued to function well in my absence.

Close friend and managing partner, Joe Garcia, visited and said my salary would continue unabated. That provided great but only temporary relief. What we didn't discuss was something Joe and I both knew; if I wasn't able to pull my weight when I returned it was at best a temporary solution.

I worked for one of the largest and most prestigious lobbying and public relations firms in Lansing, a coveted job. But not unlike the game of baseball I dearly love, you had to produce daily. If you didn't, there was always someone ready to take your place in the lineup.

Adding to my anxiety, I learned a number of purported friends had contacted the owner of the firm to see if any help was needed "just until Mike gets back." Left unsaid, but clearly implied, was that if Mike didn't return they would like to be considered when the search began for his permanent replacement. And if that search was undertaken sooner rather than later, so be it. "I understand there is a good chance Mike won't be back, or if he does return he'll never be as productive as he once was. Always loved Mike, but life goes on. No need for the business to suffer."

Politics is a cutthroat business, only now the blade was at my throat. In only a moment I could be nothing more than an afterthought.

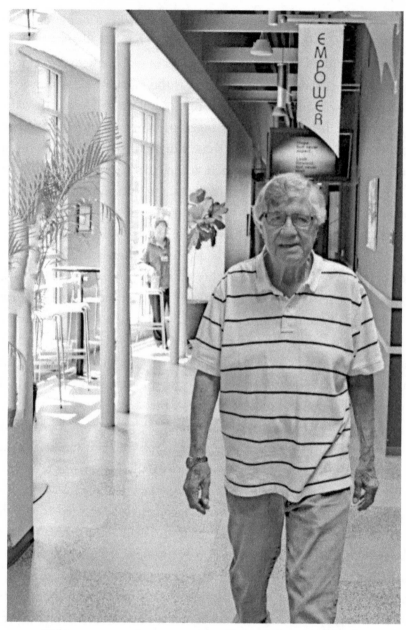

Walking was a part of my new regimen. Photo courtesy of Rod Weaver.

Walking was part of my new regimen; ten minutes at first, then gradually increasing. Ten minutes? I scoffed at ten minutes. I could easily do more than that. To my humbling surprise, at least at first, ten minutes proved to be more than an adequate goal.

My first appointment with Dr. James was scheduled for a few weeks after my discharge. I only knew him from his daily rounds in the hospital. I was fond of his frank delivery of medical news. There was no misunderstanding his assessment of my condition, no shades of gray when he spoke, no searching for purpose and intent in his message. He was friendly, though, and had a sense of humor. Once he discovered I didn't quiver at his abruptness and could handle, even appreciate, his straight-from-the shoulder brand of medicine, he warmed and gradually allowed his wit to surface.

Dr. Michael James, I learned, was a headliner in the highly-regarded Thoracic Cardiovascular Institute (TCI). A friend worked as a fundraiser for Ingham Medical Center, the hospital where I stayed and the home field for TCI. He told me TCI was the big draw for raising money, and that Mike James was the superstar of TCI.

Dr. James informed me I was being assigned to a rehabilitation program associated with his group's practice. When I voiced a concern that I was not all that confident in my ability to physically exert myself beyond walking, he looked me in the eye and uttered words that not only drove my rehabilitation, but the next several years of my life: "It's okay to sweat again."

Once I started the rehab I learned he was right. Not only was it okay to sweat again, but it felt good. No longer was I infirmed. I grew up playing sports; had the good fortune to play for coaches who believed strongly in conditioning; and conditioning meant pushing yourself. In rehab, under the watchful eye of Mary Ann Bull, I rediscovered the joy of sweating again.

A week or so before I had my heart attack, Jud Heathcote, head basketball coach at Michigan State University, also had one. While his heart problems got a little more publicity than mine, we both were assigned to the same rehab program. An icon of college basketball and a celebrity in his own right, Jud—as anyone who knows him will testify—

has a great, refined, and sometimes ribald sense of humor. And it didn't take long for it to surface.

My first rehab class came on the day following a Detroit Lions loss when their usually dependable field goal kicker, Eddie Murray, had missed three. Just before we climbed on our respective workout machines, Jud pulled me aside.

"Guess who I just saw outside the hospital?" he said, deadpan, no sign of tomfoolery.

"Who?" I asked, thrilled at individual attention from the legendary coach.

"Eddie Murray."

"No kidding," I responded, not knowing he was pulling my leg.

"I said, 'Eddie, how ya' doin'? He said, 'I dunno'. Can't kick."

I had a good laugh. As it turned out, Jud was not only the master of the one-liner, but his mischievous (albeit adult) sense of humor could also seize control of a serious moment and transform it into sheer hilarity.

In addition to the physical exertion on the machines where we all learned it was okay to sweat again, the rehab program included interaction with a cadre of other health professionals, primarily dieticians and social workers. The problem was our new tutors were all young, in their early twenties. Jud was in his late fifties, I was forty. They frequently addressed us in a sing-song fashion, not unlike the kind of voice invoked when talking to children. "This is what weee can have for breakfast. Won't that be delicious?" After our initial session with the dietician, Jud muttered to me on the way out, "I got underwear older than her."

The social worker meant well. She urged us to structure our lives so as to avoid tension. Keeping things bottled-up was not in our best interest. We all needed to have someone we could talk to, she said, someone with whom we could vent our frustrations. It was probably solid advice but was totally lost in the fact that the person delivering the message was barely out of college. It was difficult to look beyond the age differential. And I couldn't fathom Jud asking an official during a game, "Could I just have a moment to compose myself?" Serenity, I knew from following MSU basketball for a number of years, was not one of his strengths.

In our group was also a minister, a genuinely nice man. But he didn't find Jud's sometimes bawdy comments nearly as funny as I did.

Finally, just as the rehab program was coming to a close, we had a memorable counseling session devoted to resuming sex. The social worker spoke convincingly about the dangers of mixing alcohol and sex, or over-exertion, or over-indulgence. At one point, in an attempt to assist the obviously young and uncomfortable social worker, the minister spoke up, indicating he was drawing from his years of experience counseling couples.

"Fellas," he said slowly, assuming a paternal tone of voice and nodding his head knowingly, "sometimes you just can't jump in there. You have to hug 'em and kiss 'em first." Jud looked at me and rolled his eyes. I had all I could do to stifle a laugh. But then, to my delight – and the other guys in the class – Jud decided to press the matter.

Straight-faced, and without the slightest hint that his concern was anything but genuine, Jud informed the uneasy social worker: "It's been years since the wife and I have had sex without her dressed in some kind of leather and me with a paddle in my hand. Is it all right if we just pick up where we left off?"

She turned crimson and fumbled with a response that suggested it would be better if he approached sex with caution, and not get too excited, at least at first. At that point I had to leave the room.

The rehab was a success. I did sweat again. I resumed playing softball with my buddies the following summer, and even made a few contributions to the team. Key to the ritual of softball is stopping for a cold one to rehash the game, in our case at Moriarty's Pub, our team sponsor. While I never had more than two beers, those after-the-game gatherings with the guys were important. Lying in the hospital months earlier I didn't know if I would ever experience them again.

Walking became boring. I began to jog. Exercise was now a challenge; it was fun again. I even ran in a few five-mile events. I never finished with the real runners, but I didn't finish last either. Buttressed by the sage counsel of Dr. Michael James, I was sweating again, and it felt great.

I badgered Dr. James relentlessly about returning to work. He seemed unfazed. I sensed this was not his initial encounter with an obsessed patient. But then, I'm sure to get me off his back, he offered to order a stress test. If I did well he would consider a return to work. The only thing that stood between me and leaving the daytime people to fend for themselves was a treadmill. No matter how daunting that treadmill appeared when I arrived for the stress test, there was no way it was going to best me.

I did well.

After a frank conversation with Dr. James regarding diet, alcohol consumption, exercise, and the importance of rest, on November 5, forty-three days after my heart attack, I returned to work.

To my delight, or increasing anxiety, the needs of the clients I dealt with had been addressed. My partners covered for me in grand fashion.

Like Dr. James, my managing partner, Joe Garcia, lacks the finesse of an international diplomat but never delivers a message that is misinterpreted. Shortly after I appeared in the office, Joe and I had a brief but blunt conversation. He was assuming I was back - at full strength. There would be no special accommodations. No training wheels. If I needed something, it was up to me to say so. That did wonders for my anxiety and morale. No special treatment. I was not indispensable, but I was back in the lineup. All those good friends who inquired about my health and envisioned themselves holding forth from my desk would have to wait. Not unlike Tim Finnegan, the besotted corpse feted in the Irish dance hall tune "Finnegan's Wake," I just winked.

People treated me differently. I was never a particularly influential or beloved figure in the Capitol. Nevertheless, upon encountering me for the first time since the heart attack, a number of people, men included, hugged me. Thankfully, the callous nature that hovers over the political arena quickly resumed and the hugging stopped.

Every legislature runs for two years, just as each congress runs for two years. All bills not acted on by December 31 in an even-numbered year automatically die and must be reintroduced the following legislative session. This was 1984.

The time between Election Day in November and the last session of the legislative body in December is known as *lame-duck*. It is a particularly volatile time on the legislative calendar. Anything can happen, and frequently does. *Lame-duck* is a stressful period, not to mention it usually involves long hours and an occasional all-night session.

Only weeks earlier I was on my back in a hospital, a serious heart attack survivor. Now I was in the middle of the most stressful period of the year in my job. No easing gently back into the daily schedule. On the contrary, any sign of indecision or diminished physical capacity, the wolves quickly cut the tentative out from the rest of the herd. Fortunately, I was too busy to dwell on the dangers to my heart. I performed well and was even instrumental in securing passage of a bill my firm had all but determined doomed.

Joe came down to my office and delivered a ten-second speech that made it all worthwhile. "We never thought we'd get that bill. But we did. It made for a nice end to the year. Glad you're back."

The political arena can at times be a bare-knuckled, back-alley brawl. I was back, tired and bearing some scars, but able to enjoy that special feeling when the team did well and knowing you contributed. Trudging back to the office, the legislature in adjournment for the year, I thought of Dr. James and his learned counsel. There may have been a chill in the December air, but professionally I was sweating again. It felt great.

Dr. Michael James:

It has always been my goal to return the heart attack patient back to their previous life style without restrictions if I feel it is safe. I tell them if something is going to happen it's just as likely to happen if you are sitting at home worrying about your condition or back "doing your thing". We always discuss the warning signs and it is almost predictable that if further ischemia is going to occur it usually presents as the same initial symptom; i.e. Mike's initial symptom was jaw discomfort rather than chest discomfort. Then we either need to intervene with mechanical revascularization or additional meds.

Mike was back, had rejoined his firm and was doing well. Apart from Mike and his family, no one was happier than me.

CHAPTER EIGHT

Heart Disease and the Twentieth Century:

Progress and Politics

"Healthy citizens are the greatest asset a country can have."
—WINSTON CHURCHILL

Mike Ranville:

It would all be linked forever in the annals of cardiac history: two heart attacks incurred by two United States presidents, two faulty diagnoses, and two attempts to influence the news surrounding the heart attacks for political purposes.

While they were thirty-two years apart, events surrounding the heart attacks of both President Warren G. Harding in 1923, and President Dwight D. Eisenhower in 1955, were amazingly similar. An erroneous diagnosis hovered over both, and, for less than admirable reasons, in both cases the public was not accurately informed of the condition of their president.

Warren G. Harding

In the summer of 1923, while in Alaska on a political trip, President Harding complained of stomach pain. With him on the trip was close friend, homeopathic trained Dr. Charles Sawyer, who informed the accompanying press that the president's discomfort could be traced to tainted crabmeat. Shortly after his ship arrived in Seattle, Harding nearly collapsed from weakness. As he traveled on to San Francisco, the discomfort continued, but still he refused assistance, even while walking unsteadily from his limousine to the hotel.

Befitting the stature of the patient, prominent physicians in the Bay Area were summoned to Harding's bedside. Among those attending him was the President of the American Medical Association, Dr. Ray Lyman Wilbur[8].

The symptoms screamed heart attack: chest pain radiating down the arms, particularly the left arm, several attacks of indigestion, most often at night, accompanied by pain and a feeling of distress, breathing difficulties, again at night, chronic weakness.

The consensus diagnosis, however, was a gall bladder attack. Four days later, August 2, 1923, Warren Gamaliel Harding, the twenty-ninth President of the United States, died.

Questions surrounding Harding's death surfaced immediately, needless questions that only fueled an uninformed public's predisposition to readily embrace conspiracy theories. A President of the United States, an office that could and should command the most sophisticated and competent medical treatment, died suddenly. There had to be a valid reason.

Compared to the satellite-driven immediacy of today, news in 1923 tip-toed around the globe. The sudden death of a President, however, is still earth-shattering. Absent information to the contrary, coverage gaps are filled by a public perception that quickly shifts into overdrive. The death of President Harding was of sufficient import to further hasten that process.

---

8   Wilbur, a staunch Republican, would later be appointed by Herbert Hoover to serve as Secretary of the Interior.

There were a number of troubling factors. Though none were singularly alarming, taken together they raised a disturbing scenario:

- No one present—none of Harding's family, friends or staff, none of the prominent physicians attending him—could agree on a time of death: 7:10 p.m., 7:20 p.m., 7:30 p.m. were all offered.
- Accounts varied widely as to who was in the room when Harding died. No one could be sure.
- There was no agreement on the cause of death, only a general belief on the part of the hastily assembled medical team that it was heart related—perhaps a stroke—all made worse by rumors of ptomaine poisoning purportedly contracted days earlier in Vancouver. But releasing a statement that didn't enjoy the concurrence of all the attending physicians would have raised questions regarding the consensus diagnosis of gall bladder.

An autopsy surely would have resolved the dilemma. But, at the direction of Harding's wife, Florence—the president referred to her as "the Duchess"—no autopsy was performed. Inexplicably, within an hour of his death, again at her direction, he was prepared for his casket. The next morning that casket was whisked off to Washington, D.C.

Long before Harding's death, rumors abounded that he was too infirmed to function as president and the country was really being run by "the Duchess." A sudden death, left unexplained, only deepened those concerns as the news traveled across the country.

Not surprisingly, bizarre theories quickly surfaced. Suicide? But why? Murder? By whom and for what reason?

This was the death of a President, a significant moment at the time, and for history as well. Sloppy at best is a generous characterization of how it was handled.

Accurate information released in a timely fashion could have mitigated many of the burgeoning conspiracy theories. But given the misdiagnosis and subsequent swatting aside of obvious problems with the heart, accuracy would have translated into acknowledging physician error. Allowing conspiracy theories to flourish appeared preferable to conceding and defending poor medical judgment.

Dwight D. Eisenhower

Dwight David Eisenhower was a complicated man, mentally and physically. While his life is characterized by rare accomplishment, he suffered a number of chronic health maladies, mostly in silence. His heart attack in 1955, and the manner in which the public was kept informed of his condition, played a significant role in shaping public perception of heart disease[9].

Far from the easy smile Americans came to know during World War II, especially in the days leading up to and immediately following D-Day, and far from the wide grin that adorned the "I Like Ike" campaign material seven years later, Eisenhower had a volcanic temper. Allegedly he had severe temper tantrums as a child and adult. Growing up in Kansas, if things didn't go his way or he was particularly frustrated, he was known to bang his head on a tree. While he learned to manage the tantrums, they never really left him throughout his adult life, including his time in the White House.

Kay Summersby, his driver and close companion during the war, noted several instances of Ike's volatile temper, frequently over what appeared to be a trivial matter. On one occasion he erupted when the coffee was cold; on another when his brand of cigarettes was leaked to a reporter. The outbursts were accompanied by significant increases in blood pressure.

Bryce Harlow, one of President Eisenhower's speech writers and a favored staff member, recalls the President exploding at him for making minor changes to a speech that had already been approved.

Ike was beset with stomach problems throughout his life. Following graduation from West Point in 1915, records indicate that with each new

---

9   For a thorough, riveting and eloquent account of President Eisenhower's heart attack, see Clarence G. Lasby's, *Eisenhower's Heart Attack: How Ike Beat Heart Disease and Held on to the Presidency*.

assignment a different medical team would attempt (unsuccessfully as it turned out), to determine the cause of his ailing stomach. Periodically he would "give himself up" to doctors and enter a hospital for a lengthy stay to determine "once and for all" the source of his indigestion. But it didn't disappear.

With each of those stays doctors recommended he cease or severely curtail smoking, which he attempted to do. Moreover, his schedule allowed for little exercise and his diet was particularly high in starches.

Wherever he was stationed, there was a history of treating his abdominal discomfort. On more than one occasion he was told his problems stemmed from stress, nervousness, overwork, and lack of exercise. There was no question the assignments he was given throughout his entire military career were stressful, up to and including D-Day, June 6, 1944. The final days of the war proved especially hectic. Physical discomfort notwithstanding, Ike was adamant that his personal constitution and rugged frontier upbringing equipped him to handle any physical or emotional barrier placed in his path.

He came by his well-publicized love of golf naturally. Early in life he imagined a career as a professional athlete, the specific sport would be determined later. But a sprained knee ended all such hopes. He did enjoy success on the playing fields of West Point; his gridiron play even attracted the eloquent pen of Grantland Rice. With his professional athletic career doomed by the knee injury, he turned to less strenuous pursuits and took up golf.

On numerous occasions during the war, at the request of Army Chief of Staff George C. Marshall, Ike's wife Mamie was treated by Army physician Howard McCrum Snyder. After the war when Mamie's health became a concern and she was hospitalized in Boone, Iowa, Ike finally met Dr. Snyder. So began the relationship that would eventually take Dr. Howard Snyder to President Eisenhower's bedside on September 23, 1955.

Mamie quickly stabilized. Snyder accompanied Ike to a speaking engagement in Chicago where the Army doctor treated his new patient for a sore throat. The two then journeyed to Washington, D.C., where Ike testified at a congressional hearing. Again, Snyder treated Ike, this time for a sinus infection.

Shortly thereafter, Snyder helped Ike through a severe case of bronchitis that bordered on pneumonia. He ordered Eisenhower hospitalized for ten days. While in the hospital General Eisenhower learned he had been promoted to Army Chief of Staff.

Dr. Snyder was quickly appointed to a small advisory group, an appointment that conveniently translated into personal physician to Ike and Mamie, a post he retained for the next twenty years. Never far from his famous patients' side, he attended Ike during his tenure as President of Columbia University in New York, while heading SHAPE (Supreme Headquarters of Allied Powers in Europe) in France, and eventually to the White House.

Ike's Heart Attack

"I found a shocking misdiagnosis in the crucial hours after the heart attack. Dr. Snyder mistook a coronary thrombosis for a gastro-intestinal problem, waited for ten hours before he recognized his mistake and called for help, and conducted an unremitting cover-up of his error for the rest of his life."
—CLARENCE G. LASBY, *EISENHOWER'S HEART ATTACK*

On July 2, 1955, Senate Majority Leader Lyndon Johnson, a three-pack-a-day smoker, suffered a heart attack. Likely it would have been the top story of the year in Washington, save for President Eisenhower's heart attack slightly less than three months later.

Of all the heart attacks of the twentieth century, understandably none received more notoriety than that what befell Dwight D. Eisenhower, the 34th President of the United States. Sadly, despite the impact it had on the world, particularly the United States, the nature and severity of the heart attack was under-reported to the public, and for less than noble motives.

On September 23, 1955, President Eisenhower, age sixty-five, complained of growing discomfort while playing a round of golf in Denver, Colorado. He played twenty-seven holes that day.

The President was a heavy smoker. Like the majority of military personnel during World War II, General Eisenhower took advantage of free cigarettes from the tobacco companies, the same free cigarettes that would hook an entire generation on the deadly product. Further, he arguably had the most stressful job in the world. His heart attack occurred at the height of the cold war, a time when tension-filled thrust-and-parry with Russia was the daily substance of foreign policy.

Throughout his adult life, Eisenhower was plagued by severe indigestion. The President determined the discomfort was just another upset stomach so he took some Milk of Magnesia. When that didn't help, his personal physician, now Major General Howard Snyder, was summoned. General Snyder found a hypertensive President with an elevated blood pressure of 160/120.

The treatment at the time for Ike's symptoms was a hefty dose of morphine. Morphine not only addressed the pain but also functioned as a vasodilator that relaxed blood vessels and lowered pulmonary pressure. He was also given amyl nitrate to relax the arteries in the heart, and Heparin, a blood thinner. Aspirin, a mainstay of treatment today because of its anticoagulant properties, had yet to be identified as the simple but effective blood thinner of choice.

The President was also diaphoretic—sweaty and cold—another common symptom in patients experiencing a heart attack. Snyder recommended that Ike's wife, Mamie, crawl into bed with him to relieve his growing anxiety.

Incredulous as it may seem, it took nearly twenty-four hours before an EKG was ordered, and somewhere between ten and twenty-four hours before his symptoms subsided. He eventually was taken to Fitzsimons Army Hospital in Denver where an EKG revealed an anterior wall myocardial infarction. There was damage to the pumping chamber of the heart. President Eisenhower had indeed suffered a heart attack.

Bed rest for a month was prescribed. He was also kept out of Washington for an additional seven weeks. And while difficult to imagine, the President of the United States, the acknowledged leader of the free world, had no communication with his cabinet for three weeks. His treatment reflected the state of cardiac care in 1955.

The Eisenhower and Harding heart attacks warrant consideration for two reasons. First, they underscore that heart problems in general, and heart attacks in particular, can happen to anyone, even the leader of the free world. Eisenhower's in particular emphasizes to heart attack victims of today that the sooner an accurate diagnosis can be conducted, the sooner treatment can begin. The swiftness of care delivered in the minutes and hours immediately following a heart attack is crucial to saving the life of the victim, not to mention the quality of life that follows.

A review of Eisenhower's heart attack, and immediate treatment, suggest Ike was lucky, and the heartbeat that would have made Richard Nixon the 35th President of the United States was closer to not beating than the public was led to believe.

The question contemplated then, and that lingers today—could Nixon have beaten Adlai Stevenson in the 1956 presidential race – may have driven decisions affecting not only the speed of Eisenhower's real or perceived return to full command of the country, but also the nature of the information released to the public regarding the severity of his condition. In retrospect, history would surely read different today had Richard Nixon or Adlai Stevenson become the 35th president of the United States in 1956, not to mention the individual who would have assumed office in 1969.

Significant to the public persona of President Eisenhower as he recovered in Fitzsimons Army Hospital in Denver was the image planted in the public mind by advertising man Rosser Reeves[10] three years earlier during the 1952 presidential campaign. Ike was depicted as forthright, strong yet friendly. In order to foster the perception of strength, he didn't

---

10   Reeves is believed to be the model for Don Draper of the successful television program *Mad Men*.

wear his customary glasses. Maintaining that carefully-crafted image was critical to the upcoming 1956 election.

When the President of the United States becomes incapacitated, it creates a ripple effect.

When Eisenhower was sworn into office on January 20, 1953, the Dow Jones Industrial average was 288. By September 23, 1955, the day of the heart attack, that figure had climbed to 487, a 69 percent increase. Time magazine attributes the impressive growth to a belief that "...President Eisenhower would be elected for a second term in 1956 and the U.S, economic boom would continue unhindered by any political changes."[11]

Ike's heart attack occurred late in the day on Friday, September 23, 1955. Despite the dearth of information out of Denver, when the market opened the following Monday the Dow Jones average plunged thirty-two points, a 6.5 percent drop. The total paper loss for the day was $14 billion, the worst decline the New York Stock Exchange had seen since the crash on October 29, 1929.

Presidents and their health weigh heavy across the entire spectrum of America. Given that impact, accurate information, good or bad, is crucial. In Eisenhower's case not only was the medical diagnosis mishandled, but there also was a massage of medical bulletins released out of Denver regarding the President's condition.

Once it was determined that Ike had indeed suffered a heart attack, renowned cardiologist Paul Dudley White was summoned.

Partisan politics can be brutal. Congress is replete with stories of members being wheeled on to the floor to vote when they hardly had the strength to answer roll call. Once their vote is cast, they are wheeled out just as quickly for fear the public might ask what price victory? Was the issue worth retrieving the ailing lawmaker from a hospital bed just to cast a vote? If the vote proved to be pivotal, the answer would be a resounding yes, accompanied by a press release indicating the courageous lawmaker

---

11   "Wall Street: Black Monday," <u>Time Magazine</u>, 10 October 1955,

insisted on making the journey to the floor, swatting aside personal discomfort to gallantly perform a sworn duty.

Even in the early stages of Ike's recovery, no matter the toll on his personal health, there were political partisans who urged him to seek re-election. At stake, after all, was control of the government for the next four years; thousands of patronage jobs, thousands of lucrative government contracts, a political philosophy markedly different from the Democrats in general and Adlai Stevenson in particular.

The country did indeed "like Ike." He was the odds-on favorite to win the upcoming presidential election. It was important for the American people to know their President could withstand the rigors of a national campaign; a public perception of weakness or lack of vitality on the part of Ike could translate into a loss of votes. What information did reach the people regarding his health was crafted to reassure voters that he was capable of mounting a vigorous defense of his presidency, and fully equipped for the demanding task of running the country for the next four years. He had to appear as the strong, vibrant leader. And so the communiqués out of Denver were fashioned accordingly.

Unlike Dr. Howard Snyder, the President's personal physician who worked closely with those encouraging Ike to run, Dr. Paul Dudley White was far more cautious. Time notes his response to a query of whether or not the president was physically able to run with, "Oh yes." However, later that same day on a show with popular television host Dave Garroway, White cautiously pointed out, "If I were in his shoes I wouldn't want to run again, having seen the strain[12]."

White's candor did not endear him to the political partisans. While placing the interest of his patient first, White inadvertently was cast in the role of villain.

Like Warren Harding years earlier, information, important and trivial, was carefully managed.

---

12   Ibid.

Medical bulletins regarding Eisenhower's condition were carefully structured. Only Mrs. Eisenhower, Vice President Nixon, and White House Chief of Staff Sherman Adams were fully informed of the complete diagnosis. Fearing a leak if the those in the know group was expanded, other government officials did not even learn of the heart attack until twelve hours after the EKG; not the Secretary of State, not the Secretary of Defense, not the Attorney General.

In an effort to give the appearance that full disclosure was the order of the day, the public was inundated with trivial information. Such details as Ike wearing pajamas with five gold stars on the collar, the frequency of bowel movements, the detection of a slight fever after taking the temperature rectally, and other intimate particulars of the nursing care he received, had the intended effect of prompting criticism of too much information, of an invasion of the President's privacy. The public was uneasy; Ike deserved greater respect. All of which afforded a convenient justification to withhold and control information regarding the president's true condition.

In 1919, President Woodrow Wilson suffered a severe stroke that left him incapacitated until the end of his presidency in 1921, an event that became one of the great crises in presidential succession[13]. During the last eight months of Wilson's presidency, the only people with access to him were his wife, secretary, and physician, raising valid concerns regarding who was really running the country. With the pending presidential race hovering, the political partisans were well aware of mistakes by Woodrow Wilson's administration.

Time Magazine, under the direction of its founder and editor-in-chief, conservative Republican Henry Luce, buttressed the effort to portray a strong and vibrant Eisenhower and underscored all was functioning well under Vice President Richard Nixon, the carefully chosen next-in-command.

---

13   Joan Schlimgen, "Woodrow Wilson—Strokes and Denial," The University of Arizona Health Sciences Library, (23 January 2012)

In a lengthy article two weeks after Ike's heart attack, Time stressed that Nixon had been carefully groomed by the President to step in immediately should events dictate. The article also pointed out that Nixon was keeping Ike informed, and that the President was definitely in command of the ship of state.[14]

Ike's Chief of Staff, Sherman Adams, spent most of the week with the President at Fitzsimons Hospital. He would fly back to Washington for a Friday Cabinet meeting presided over by Vice President Nixon. To the consternation of the partisans, Adams acquired the moniker of "acting president."

Three weeks after the heart attack Time ran an article portraying a healing and vibrant Eisenhower, not only attending to matters of state while conferring with Vice President Nixon and Secretary of State John Foster Dulles, but also enjoying tapes from his grandchildren. His mind was active and he also loved the mental gymnastics with an Army nurse who brought in quiz books the two drew on to challenge each other[15].

Eisenhower's triumphant departure for Washington finally arrived when it was determined he could execute a vigorous walk to the plane.

An old axiom of politics, perception is reality, was alive and well that fall of 1955.

Heart Disease—Public Perception Then and Now

During the intervening thirty-two years between the Harding and Eisenhower heart attacks, heart disease continued to dominate as the number one killer in the United States. In many cases it was sudden death, a heart attack, often accompanied by a comment such as, "But I just talked to him this morning!"

It was not uncommon for a movie or television drama to show a man—and usually it was a man, even though heart disease is a leading cause of death in women—consumed by the emotions of the moment, gripping his chest and falling to the ground. We all knew he just had a

---

14   "The Vice-Presidency: The Acting Captain," <u>Time Magazine</u>, 10 October 10 1955,
15   "The Presidency: The Time Of Healing," <u>Time Magazine</u>, 17 October 1955,

heart attack. Temperamental actors quickly learned it was a quick and convenient way for maligned writers to kill off a character.

Heart attack, myocardial infarction, coronary thrombosis—it goes by many names. But it can strike at any moment, and does not defer to fame or fortune.

Lasby recounts the fascinating and prescient paper delivered in 1772 to the Royal College of Physicians by King George III's physician William Heberden. Heberden used the term "angina pectoris." So accurate was his description of "angina pectoris," that Heberden's description was still in use in 1972, two hundred years later.

From Heberden's 1772 report: "They that are afflicted with it, are seized while they are walking, more especially if it be up hill, and soon after eating with a painful and most disagreeable sensation in the breast, which seems as if it would extinguish life, if it were to increase or continue, but the moment they stand still, all this uneasiness vanishes." He goes on to point out that those most vulnerable to experiencing angina pectoris are "males, especially those as have passed their fiftieth year."

Heberden wrote that after the discomfort in the breast has continued for a year or more, standing still no longer sends the pain away. Frequently it begins occurring at night or when the patient is lying down, especially on the left side. He didn't shy from the sudden death aspects of angina pectoris: "If no accidents intervene, but the disease goes on to its height, the patients all suddenly fall down, and perish almost immediately." He also recognized the role of emotion and stress, "It (angina pectoris) is increased by disturbance of the mind."

Heberden observes, "Wine and spirituous liquors, and opium afford considerable relief." Almost 200 years later President Eisenhower was given a hefty dose of morphine following his heart attack.

Lasby cites other observations from the eighteenth century.

The role played by passion and emotion was recorded when famed surgeon John Hunter was fatally stricken after a heated exchange with the Board of Governors of his hospital.

Another crucial contribution followed the discovery of a substance as hard as a rock during an examination of the arteries of a deceased person. When falling plaster from the ceiling was ruled out as a cause, the arteries were described as little more than bony canals.

While little was forthcoming in the way of relief for the "disagreeable sensation in the breast," it steadfastly remained in the public eye, primarily because of the riveting pain and sudden death.

Not all the forthcoming information proved useful. While genes were suspected as a leading culprit in heart disease no direct link was established. That didn't deter a prominent Cleveland physician, though. In 1932 he offered his 'thinning out the herd" theory that heart disease was the natural consequence of the aging process, and that deterioration of the arteries appeared to be nature's favored way of eliminating those whose biological responsibilities had been fulfilled.

In 1905, heart disease replaced tuberculosis and pneumonia as the leading killer in the United States, a position it has yet to relinquish. Few families have escaped its impact. While detection has improved over the years, the medical community originally developed little in the way of care or prevention. There was a school of thought that believed one's cardiac fate, good or bad, had been determined long ago, probably before birth. But there were others, and their numbers were steadily growing, who felt a diseased heart could be treated, that it was not an automatic death sentence. While elimination of heart disease was not realistic, the incapacitating effects could be tempered.

In 1945 the American Heart Association (AHA) was formed. Chief among the group's initial contributions was their annual conference, a forum for the exchange of ideas and research, and their highly-regarded, research-oriented American Heart Journal.

The AHA also recruited laymen to raise funds for research and financing sorely needed campaigns to increase public awareness of heart disease. One sobering statistic drove their early efforts: while 185,000 Americans died of cancer in 1945, 658,000 died of heart problems.

President Franklin D. Roosevelt lent the prestige of his office to fight polio, the disease that afflicted him, by supporting the highly popular March of Dimes campaign. President Eisenhower did not use his bully pulpit to support heart disease prevention efforts. When asked to assume the honorary post of President of the American Heart Association, a position many felt would significantly increase resources to combat heart disease, the President demurred and recommended his brother Dr. Milton Eisenhower.

Conspicuous by its absence in the fight against heart disease was government, the weight and influence of the federal government in particular. Enter Albert and Mary Lasker whose efforts were instrumental in creating and nurturing awareness of the dreaded killer.

Albert Lasker, who rightfully enjoyed the moniker "Father of American Advertising," was well known beyond advertising circles. He was an early owner of the Chicago Cubs and influential in bringing the team to its current home, storied Wrigley Field. Following the Black Sox scandal, where eight members of the Chicago White Sox were accused of consorting with gamblers to throw the 1919 World Series, he authored and advanced the so-called Lasker Plan, calling for reforms that led to creation of the office of Commissioner of Baseball, and invested strong authority in the position. Many felt the Lasker Plan saved the great American pastime.

Lasker was the first to apply modern day advertising techniques to politics. He successfully lent his considerable talent to the 1920 Warren G. Harding presidential campaign. Harding's image pervaded newsreels, billboards, and newspapers, leading him and running-mate Calvin Coolidge to a convincing victory over Democratic hopefuls James C. Cox and Franklin D. Roosevelt. As a result, Albert Lasker enjoyed a commanding presence while navigating the corridors of power in Washington, D.C.

In 1942, he sold his agency, Lord and Thomas, for a considerable profit and, along with his third wife Mary, set out on a life of philanthropy in general and improving the country's health in particular. They were instrumental in promoting and expanding the National Institutes of

Public Health. They also founded and endowed the Lasker Award that recognized and rewarded leading scientists and researchers.

During his tenure as an advertising executive Lasker devised a copywriting technique of appealing directly to an individual consumer. Ironically, that method proved highly effective in increasing sales of Lucky Strikes cigarettes, particularly among women. Smoking Luckies, he claimed, would keep them slender.

Albert and Mary Lasker were a formidable team. Armed with Albert's promotional talents and substantial checkbook, coupled with Mary's vast retinue of influential friends and an uncanny ability to move the sluggish machinery of politics and government, they turned their attention to the country's biggest killer; heart disease.

Mary Lasker was not to be outworked. She fashioned an extensive fact-sheet on heart disease, citing horrendous statistics that buttressed her case for federal involvement. Prior to her research much of the information involving heart disease was anecdotal.

The fact-sheet enjoyed wide distribution. It dominated what turned out to be lengthy and sometimes controversial congressional hearings. So thorough was her command of the subject, so complete was her recitation of the salient facts, that it drove the national discussion on heart disease for years to come. It also prompted an effort to begin keeping accurate statistics so as to adequately assess the extent of the problem.

Skeptics asked, "Should government resources be appropriated to fight heart disease and should control of research and medical funds be subject to political influence?"

"Yes!" Mary Lasker emphatically responded. Her fact-sheet invoked the appalling figure that more people were lost every year to heart disease than were killed in World War II.

Mary Lasker didn't start at the bottom. She enlisted old friend and consummate Washington insider Clark Clifford to her cause. Clifford had served FDR during the war and was currently a top advisor to President Harry Truman. She also conscripted World War II hero William "Wild

Bill" Sullivan, former head of the Office of Strategic Services[16]. Sullivan directed attention to the last war where the country spent more than a quarter of a billion dollars a day to fight the military enemy; yet a common enemy, heart disease, was allowed to go unchecked and murder 600,000 of its citizens every year. Surgeon General Dr. Leonard Steele punctuated Sullivan's comments by pointing out that delaying action translated into a death sentence for 600,000 people.

When access to President Truman via Clark Clifford was joined with a vast array of congressional contacts, Mary Lasker was the driving force behind creation of the National Heart Institute. An immediate impact of her effort was a renewed focus on diet and stress. Further, through the gathering of valuable data, the National Heart Institute[17] was able to quantify what many had feared—few homes in the country were immune from a fatal heart attack.

Ike's Infarct—2017 Version

Dr. Michael James:

Ike had his heart attack (myocardial infarction) at age sixty-five in 1955, basically the "dark ages" of cardiology. Bluntly, he was lucky. Despite the fact that he remained in bed for hours, time that delayed not only a correct diagnosis but critical treatment, he eventually returned to full activity, served a second term, and lived to age seventy-eight.

Unlike 1955, today whenever and wherever a president travels medical emergencies are anticipated, and, to the extent possible, immediate care readily available. If, for instance, Ike's infarction occurred today, and was correctly diagnosed, he would quickly be dispatched to the nearest hospital that offered a 24/7-catheterization lab where attempts would be made to open his occluded artery as soon as possible.

I distinctly recall an occasion when President Bill Clinton was scheduled to appear at Michigan State University. Preparations by the advance team ensured that one of our interventional cardiologists would remain in the

---

16   Forerunner of the Central Intelligence Agency.
17   Now known as the National Heart, Lung, and Blood Institute.

hospital from the time Air Force One landed until it departed. If the President suffered a heart attack, the offending artery could be opened immediately. Additionally, an open operating room was at the ready, as was a trauma team—not just on call, but physically in house.

Planning for a Presidential visit is obviously more extensive and complex than in 1955. The president's primary physician is an integral component of the official party. Further, anticipating and providing for medical emergencies, with an emphasis on access to the local cardiac community, are critical components of the advance team's duties. Any complaint involving discomfort above the diaphragm can be immediately assessed and an EKG generated.

Today, be it the President of the United States or John Q. Citizen, any delay in diagnosing a suspected heart problem is roundly criticized. We have embraced the philosophy that the quicker circulation can be restored the smaller the heart attack, the greater the longevity and the more productive the patient's remaining years. Or the more direct version, "time is muscle."

How would things be different today if Dwight D. Eisenhower, President of the United States, came off the golf course complaining of a general discomfort? Given his history of acute indigestion, he understandably turned to a routine remedy, and took Milk of Magnesia. But it didn't work and his personal physician was called.

The discomfort was persistent. In 2017 he would immediately be hospitalized and assigned to the Cardiac Care Unit (CCU) where his heart rate, rhythm, and blood pressure would be continuously monitored. His breathing would be made easier with nasal oxygen (oxygen tents are now in the Smithsonian). Just as in 1955, he would be placed on blood thinners and administered nitrates intravenously (amyl nitrate is never used in cardiology today) to relax the arteries in the heart. He would be given beta blockers, ace inhibitors, most likely would have a stent in his heart and be on powerful anti-platelet drugs (Plavix, Brillinta, are just a couple). A statin to lower his LDL (Low-density lipoprotein or good cholesterol) would also have been started; the lower the LDL the better—the goal is between 70 and 80.

Again, turning to Lasby's excellent account of Ike's heart attack, the president's arrhythmia was erratic. Today he would be given an anti-arrhythmic agent, more than likely lidocaine or amiodarone. Arrhythmias in 1955 were responsible for high mortality rates before CCUs. Ike's luck held, though; he did not develop a more serious life-threatening arrhythmia, as it is doubtful a defibrillator was at hand, and CPR was not universally known at that time.

Absolute bed rest was ordered, to the point that he was not allowed to use the commode. And that bed rest was prolonged. Today, as soon as the rhythm problem is addressed, patients are up and walking and out of the CCU in three days. They are assigned to a step-down unit and prepared for discharge in five to seven days.

While Ike's hospital stay was close to six weeks, today he would be out of the hospital and starting cardiac rehab in six weeks.

Further, the blood thinner Coumadin was the only medicine Ike was on. Today he would be on a beta-blocker, ace inhibitor, statin, an antiplatelet, and likely an anti-arrhythmic drug.

Ike's follow-up treatment included an EKG, chest x-ray, and a physical exam. The x-ray revealed "a small bulge at the apex of the heart," most likely an aneurysm, which is a harboring place for further arrhythmias and increases the risk of sudden death in heart attack patients.

In 1955, there were no tools to evaluate the coronary anatomy and nothing but the physical exam to evaluate the function of the left ventricle. During the physical exam an erratic rhythm was documented and Ike was placed on Quinidine, a drug not used today due to documented dangers of sudden death.

He certainly would have an evaluation of his left ventricle and a determination made regarding the existence of other areas of ischemia, a restriction of blood supply. An Echocardiogram and a nuclear stress test would be administered. If his nuclear scan showed any evidence of ischemia he would be given a stent or maybe even a coronary artery bypass graft (CABG).

Assuming his arrhythmia was multiple ventricular contractions, which they most likely were, and assuming he would have had at least three in a row—both logical assumptions—he would be recommended for an Implantable Cardioverter Defibrillator (ICD), that basically watches the heart for abnormal rhythms. If they occur the ICD will administer a series of shocks starting low and increasing in voltage if the lesser discharges don't abort or correct the abnormal life threatening rhythm.

The media would surely conduct an extensive discussion of ICDs; their purpose, their benefits, and, most assuredly, their drawbacks. In the "nothing is off limits" political arena of 2017, an ICD in a President would surely become partisan fodder. The opposing party would ask. "What if the ICD discharged in the middle of a national defense emergency?" Would it impact the ability to render a clear-headed decision?" Conversely, "What if there was no ICD to discharge during a national defense emergency, and one was needed?"

Ike made an impressive recovery. Despite a misdiagnosis, no monitoring of his rhythm, no medications to decrease mortality, no cardiac catheterization, and no ICD, he soldiered on. He won a second term and presided over, among other things, creation of the monumental interstate highway system and integration of the Little Rock schools. He died at age seventy-eight with his respected page in history intact. By all accounts he enjoyed his post-presidential years and lived well. He played golf almost daily, fully enjoying his open invitation to the most prestigious golf club in the United States, Augusta National. He even had his own cottage on the grounds. There is a productive life after a heart attack.

Another explanation, perhaps just as valid, is that the good Lord looked over the shoulder of President Dwight D. Eisenhower throughout his life.

CHAPTER NINE:

Dick and Mike

*"There are more things in heaven and earth, Horatio,
Than are dreamt of in your philosophy"*
HAMLET, ACT 1, SCENE V

Mike Ranville:

While Dick Cheney and I hail from totally separate stations in life, have never met and differ markedly in the social resources at our disposal, the quality and availability of today's cardiac care provided to both of us was remarkably similar. We owe our lives to that care, and those that provided it. Even though we reside at opposite ends of the political spectrum, I feel a strong kinship with former Vice-President Dick Cheney. There is much we hold in common, and much for me to admire in him.

We both count strong, independent, caring women among our immediate family. We both worked in high stress jobs in the political arena – admittedly his arena was infinitely more expansive and consequential than mine, but providing for your family can be just as stressful. And we both benefited from sophisticated advancements in cardiac care not even dreamt of by the previous generation.

Unlike famous heart patients who have gone before him, Dick Cheney, to his unending credit, summoned the celebrity of his high office to draw attention to America's number one killer, and did so by opening his own medical file for all to see. Surely he was counseled not to do so, that inviting comment on his heart problems in the strident partisan atmosphere that hovers over the national political scene was tantamount to political suicide. Yet he seized the moment and heart patients everywhere, both now and in the future, reap the benefits of his courageous decision.

While Cheney's bouts with devices and personal experiences usually preceded mine, I am a heart patient who regularly follows political issues, and the participants who drive those issues. I was more than familiar with his heart problems. And, more importantly, what was done to treat those problems.

His book, *Heart*, written with Dr. Jonathan Reiner, M.D., the cardiologist who administered to his ailing heart over time, begins with a near death episode. In 2010 Dick Cheney was in end stage heart failure. "If this is dying," Cheney told himself, "it isn't all that bad." His problems had reached the point where he could not return to his beloved Wyoming due to the high altitude. A few short years later I would have a similar confrontation with my mortality. My thoughts on that night were not unlike his.

After my heart attack in 1984, I followed closely the lives of those in the news who also had heart problems: Lyndon Johnson, Bo Schembechler and Martin Sheen are three that come to mind. Their attraction was simple: they were all leading productive lives, and doing so in pressure-laden jobs.

But the heart attack victim I was drawn to most was Dick Cheney. As his career progressed, as the shadow he cast in Washington grew steadily longer, so did my interest in him.

He wasn't always a household name. But to those of us in Michigan Dick Cheney was more than just a Wyoming Congressman who rose through the ranks of House leadership and then tapped to serve as Secretary of Defense in the George H. W. Bush administration. We knew him because he was chief of staff to Gerald Ford, the only President to ever call Michigan home.

Dick Cheney moved front and center on the national scene in 2000 when he was charged by GOP Presidential candidate George W. Bush with creating a short list of names for consideration as potential running mates. Bush instead surprised the political world by casting aside the list and selecting Cheney himself for the number two post.

With Cheney as the Vice Presidential candidate on the 2000 GOP ticket, heart problems once again were inserted into the world of partisan politics. But unlike the stonewalling—the carefully controlled flow of information associated with President Eisenhower's heart problems just prior to the 1956 campaign—this time candor triumphed, because Dick Cheney and his family insisted on it.

After the announcement, concern predictably surfaced that Cheney's health problems raised serious concern that he could be residing "a heartbeat away from the presidency." Was it just routine, nothing is off limits, no holds barred, political partisanship? Or did the charges have merit?

The GOP rejoinder quickly directed attention to John Kennedy's numerous health issues, both acknowledged and rumored, and Lyndon Johnson's 1955 heart attack that occurred within days of President Eisenhower's. Nevertheless, suitability for office, real or imagined, had definitely become a campaign issue. Certainly there was much to draw on for his opponents:

- Cheney was a three-pack-a-day smoker, for 20 years.
- In 1978, at age 37, he had a heart attack.
- He had two more heart attacks, in 1984 and 1988.
- In 1988 he underwent quadruple artery bypass grafting.

There occurred yet another cardiac-related incident, but this time safely after the polls had closed.

In late November, 2000, while the country awaited results of the legal hassles surrounding the Florida recount, Vice President-elect (maybe) Cheney was going about the business of setting up a new government.

Given his years as a Washington insider, and his extensive knowledge and experience in government, presiding over the transition understandably fell to Dick Cheney. With the recount hovering, tension was palpable as Cheney worked out of a makeshift office in Tysons Corner in nearby Virginia.

George Bush and Dick Cheney did not want to repeat mistakes of the past when holdovers from previous administrations were not replaced until well into the second year. Names for key posts were being sorted; expedited background checks underway.

On November 22, after the election but before the inauguration, Cheney woke his wife Lynne, complaining of chest discomfort. While he could cite a number of false alarms over the years involving similar symptoms, he decided to be on the safe side and determined a trip to the hospital was warranted. As he learned from his first heart attack twenty-two years earlier, "When in doubt, check it out."

Preliminary tests indicated no increase in enzyme levels; that implied no damage to the heart and, hence, no heart attack. But Dr. Reiner was not satisfied and wisely recommended a catheterization, the results of which revealed a 90% blockage in one of the coronary arteries. A stent was inserted to open the damaged artery.

Of significance, subsequent blood tests showed enzyme levels were in fact elevated, increasing the likelihood that Cheney had suffered a mild heart attack.

When the announcement came from Austin, Texas, where George Bush, technically still Governor of Texas, had set up headquarters, a decision was made to go with the original diagnosis and formally announce "no heart attack." If warranted, Cheney had exacted an internal understanding the assessment could and would be immediately amended. Unlike press briefings involving Ike's heart attack 45 years earlier, any attempt to massage or control the medical bulletins in this day of instant communication would not only prove futile but inflict untold damage on the credibility of the new administration, and do so even before the oaths of office were taken.

After the Bush camp settled on the original diagnosis of no heart attack to inform their announcement, the cardiac team treating Cheney in Washington held a press conference of their own where they divulged that the enzyme levels were elevated. Critical to their choice of wording, or in this case the lack of it, the Washington cardiologists did not actually use the term heart attack.

Concerned over potential claims of being less than forthright, claims that definitely would develop legs, the Cheney family insisted on another press conference. Again, the choice of language was critical, but in this case candor prevailed. The doctors told the press, "This would be the smallest possible heart attack a person can have and still have it classified as a heart attack."

Dick Cheney's health problems moved to the back page of the paper, giving way to the more pressing story of who would be the next president. On December 12, 2000, the U.S. Supreme Court allowed Florida Secretary of State Katherine Harris's certification of George Bush as the state's winner to stand, giving him one more than the required 270 electoral votes needed to become President. On January 20, 2001, George Walker Bush was sworn in as the 43rd President of the United States. Minutes later, the most famous heart patient in the country, Richard Bruce Cheney, was officially ensconced as the new Vice President of the United States.

Despite political misgivings, I joined with heart patients everywhere to applaud the fact that one of our own boldly demonstrated to the world that heart disease was not a death sentence and we were capable of making contributions, both on the world stage and on Main Street, U.S.A.

President Eisenhower eschewed the enormous influence of his office to advance the cause of combating the nation's number one killer. Vice President Cheney spread his arms wide, seized the moment and invited all to celebrate with him the amazing advancements realized in returning heart patients to the workplace. He became a leader in the fight against heart disease, and did so by simply letting his own story tell itself.

Dick Cheney's willingness to open his medical file, including acquisition of an ICD and later a Left Ventricular Assist Device (LVAD), coupled with his willingness to candidly discuss any aspect of that medical file, blunted the partisan attacks directed at his ability to serve before they could even get started. Unlike Ike, he seized control of the issue, didn't allow the opposition to define it. He informed the public what an ICD was, how many people in everyday life were sporting them, and how it carried the potential to improve, not hamper, his performance.

Before opponents could tag him as "infirmed," he fashioned his own image of a robust vice President going about the people's business.

Cheney received the ICD during a weekend. The following Monday reporters were told that the Vice President showed up for work at 7:43 a.m., to join the President for the daily intelligence and defense briefing. President Bush joked to the press, "We were doing a few jumping jacks before you guys got here."

Vice President Dick Cheney sent the strong, clear message that he was not shying from the political battle, but the discussion regarding his health and ability to perform the duties of his office was finished before it ever became an issue. Someone else would have to watch daytime television; along with Dick Cheney us heart patients were going to work. Bring it on.

FREDDIE THOMAS

While I continued to closely monitor the cardiac health of Dick Cheney, not all heart patients are accorded the round-the-clock resources available to the Vice President. My interest leaned toward the heart patients who staff the offices, work the production lines, and teach the children—the everyday person with heart disease. Their numbers are legion. To gain a broader perspective of heart patients, Dr. James urged me to contact other heart patients. One, Freddie Thomas, stood out. Before I could make the call, Freddie and I met by chance.

We were both asked to participate in a forum of cardiologists from across the mid-west. The event was sponsored by Thoratec, maker of the Heartmate II, the LVAD sported by both Freddie and me. While I acquired my LVAD at the University of Michigan, Freddie at Henry Ford Hospital in Detroit, our experiences both before and after, were amazingly similar. It helped to know that I was not unique.

Our role in the forum was to answer questions regarding our devices, what led up to getting them and what changes, if any, in our quality of life were brought about by the LVADs. Freddie was accompanied by his wife Wilma. He is 62 years old, articulate and energetic. We hit it off immediately.

We compared notes. His heart problems started with a heart attack in November, 2001. Like so many heart patients, genes played a key role. Both his parents died of heart attacks in their sixties, while a brother died at age 28—of a heart attack.

Through the years his life slowly deteriorated. In the fall of 2013 he became a viable candidate for an LVAD. Like me, there was little quality in his life; no energy, barely able to get through the day. The slightest movement prompted shortness of breath. Freddie was wheelchair bound. Doctors could not control his skyrocketing blood pressure. "This was no way to live," he said. "I had one foot in the grave."

Earlier in life Freddie was an athlete, primarily baseball and track. Track, in particular, requires not only speed but endurance. Where once he could seemingly run forever, now the journey from one room to the next was accomplished only by stopping to rest and wait for normal breathing to resume.

"I was beyond any help until I got my LVAD," he told me. "A meeting was held to determine who would receive an LVAD. If they sent me home without one, I knew I would be dead in five months." They didn't.

In November of 2013, Freddie Thomas joined the ranks of LVAD recipients. He doesn't remember anything that happened over the next two weeks, just woke up one day and found a scar on his chest. Two weeks later he started re-hab. Once the LVAD is implanted, sitting around and watching daytime television is no longer an option.

We both agreed that family plays a critical role in the after-care. Freddie's wife Wilma, for all intents and purposes, represented his primary care. When the situation warranted, she took advantage of the hospital's reduced cost rooms available to the family of patients. On other occasions, she slept in the room with him. She would commonly stay for three days at a time, go home for a night to do laundry, sort through the mail and attend to any pressing needs involving the home. Freddie said it best, "Nobody has your back like family."

Wilma's devotion to Freddie easily qualifies her as the much-needed spouse of a heart patient. In addition to the comfort and personal support family represents, both Freddie and I learned it helps to have another set of eyes and ears when great volumes of information and instructions are thrown at you every day. Nothing, absolutely nothing, is more important to resuming a normal life than the solid foundation family provides.

Today Freddie Thomas leads a full life that bears little resemblance to the sedentary existence of the pre-LVAD days. He works out at the gym on a daily basis; in fact he gets visibly upset if circumstances come between him and his workout.

He has become an outspoken advocate of the LVAD. On occasion he is called on to talk to others, cardiologists included, regarding the transformation in his life. And he is a superb spokesman.

CHAPTER TEN:

The Tools of the Electrophysiologist

Pacemakers

Dr. Michael James:

It's interesting that the four components of the heart—the valves, the muscle or pump, the coronary arteries, and the electrical system—all work together. Yet, they can malfunction independently.

A pacemaker consists of a battery housed in a titanium can, which also holds the components that can be programmed within the device, and an electrode or electrical cord that is placed inside the chambers of the heart. A short electrical stimulus is transmitted to the endocardium (the inner layer of the heart) producing a heartbeat. Sounds simple; but it took a while to get it right.

The original device was placed in the right ventricle. It had a single electrode and two properties; one to pace the heart and one to sense the heart. So when the patient's heart rate dropped to a prescribed level, the pacer would sense it, kick in, and pace the heart until the rate increased. Then the pacemaker would shut down and continuously monitor the heart rate until needed again.

The initial pacemakers were fortunate to last two years. The electrodes often dislodged even before the patient left the hospital. They had to be repositioned, which meant opening the incision and starting over. So much for returning to a "normal life".

The older devices were subject to the hazards of external stimuli that the pacemaker would "sense" and then turn itself off. Many can recall signs in party stores and gas stations with microwave ovens warning patients with pacemakers to stay clear. Like the pacemakers, though, the microwave ovens were old. And like the pacemakers, the microwave ovens also migrated to a new generation of more sophisticated technology. Currently, a patient with a pacemaker could sit inside a microwave oven and the device would not be affected.

When I first started my Fellowship, pacemakers were in their infancy and constantly being perfected. The initial pacemakers were single chamber and not unlike a metronome. They would pace and sense, which was good for patients who experienced long pauses or complete heart blockage. But the fixed cardiac output was not good for active patients.

Enter, once again, the engineers. Their research labs produced physiologic pacemakers that sensed when the patient needed more cardiac output and then increased the heart rate appropriately. The basic sensor was a piezo electrode, comparable to a carpenter's level with a bubble in it that sensed movement up to 1/1000 of a millimeter and then sent a signal to the battery to increase the heart rate. The idea was that if a patient was walking there was movement of the large muscles in the heart that could be sensed, prompting an appropriate increase in the heart rate.

Developing a more effective pacemaker was an ongoing production.

Some of the initial challenges, apart from the obvious size of the unit, involved the ability to tell when the battery was wearing down. The most logical of indicators would be a slow decrease in heart rate that would suggest battery depletion and signal it was time to electively replace the unit.

General Electric expressed interest in entering the field of pacemakers. They promoted the notion of increasing the heart rate when the battery was wearing out. But there was an engineering gaffe. Instead of increasing the heart rate slowly, the GE device would take off at a rate of two hundred beats per minute. When patients arrived in the Emergency Room, the electrode had to be cut; hopefully the patient had an underlying heart rate.

The story of the "Pacemaker Runaway" dominated headlines across the country. General Electric took a hit. The sale of their washers, dryers, irons, refrigerators, and other items plummeted as did the price of their stock. Sadly, but understandably, GE abandoned their involvement in pacemaker production. Today, the pacemaker/defibrillator market is a multi-billion-dollar industry.

Both the market and the sophistication of the pacemakers grew appreciably. Today's pacemakers easily last eight to ten years and include multiple programmable features. Moreover, we are now pacing three chambers; the right atrium, the right ventricle, and the left ventricle.

Also, surgical technique has dramatically simplified. It now consists of a small incision below the clavicle. The electrodes are passed through the vein under the clavicle. The procedure is usually performed using local sedation with the patient awake.

My fascination with pacemakers began when I was a Fellow. I leaped at every opportunity to scrub and participate with a few of the thoracic Fellows during surgery to insert them. While at the Burns Clinic I perfected the technique.

I traveled around the country to the various manufacturers' animal labs until I was completely comfortable with both the atrial and ventricular leads.

When I returned to Lansing and TCI, I applied for surgical privileges so I could insert them. But my request was not met with universal applause. After much debate and strident opposition from the surgeons, I was able to secure privileges, but privileges only; I received no help or support from them. There was one notable exception, Dr. J. Y. Jung, who offered assistance. Sadly, his colleagues admonished him for helping me, saying I was performing implants they would normally be doing. I was, according to them, taking food off their table, and Jr. Jung's assistance to me made him a willing accomplice. Never mind what served the patient best.

To his credit, Dr. Jung responded to the criticism by telling his colleagues he was confident that I was well-versed with the science behind the devices, and, further, they had more than enough "business" with the high numbers of bypass surgeries being performed.

I became the only cardiologist in the area implanting pacemakers, performing 90 percent of the surgeries from 1980 until we recruited a full-fledged Electrophysiologist in 1994. I helped him transition from the cutdown technique of the cephalic vein to the percutaneous approach of engaging the subclavian vein.

I also trained the cardiology fellows in pacemaker implantation. Today 99% of pacemakers are implanted by cardiologists. It's not always a routine procedure. Occasionally, the subclavian vein cannot be accessed, or more commonly the cardiac vein is inadequate and the surgeon needs to place the electrode directly on the heart so a small incision is needed. Nothing insurmountable, but training is essential, especially when the unexpected occurs.

General cardiologists rarely implant devices anymore. I, however, was at the right place at the right time.

ICDs

"Given the nature and severity of your heart attack, you should no longer be with us. Statistically you are dead.
—DR. MICHAEL JAMES TO MICHAEL RANVILLE

Mike Ranville:

While I had become accustomed to, and fully appreciated, Dr. James's belief that patients should always be told the unequivocal truth regarding their condition, I was not fully prepared to learn that I had died some time ago, at least in the world of statistical probability. According to Dr. James I had outlived the probability tables: I should have died, or at a minimum, experienced another severe heart attack long ago.

I waited—in vain as it turned out—for some sign that this was a joke, nothing more than the finely-honed Dr. James sense of humor in overdrive. Delivered during a routine visit to the office, the sobering message hung there as the room turned uncomfortably silent. I searched his eyes, his expression, for a twinkle or half grin, anything that would precede a "gotcha." Nothing. He sat for a moment without speaking and let the message settle.

I was shocked. This was the first piece of bad news since the heart attack, years earlier. Had I gotten too cocky? Maybe I wasn't the poster boy for recovery that I thought. But I was feeling fine; walking, working, navigating without effort the staircases put in front of me by the world. No physical activity had been denied me due to a heart attack.

By all accounts, Dr. James continued, due to my low ejection fraction, at the very least I should be experiencing severe congestive heart failure, maybe even more. I quickly translated. I was a time bomb living on the precipice of detonation. I knew the statistics related to congestive heart failure and second heart attacks, and they did not favor the patient. For whatever reason, though, this is the first time anyone drove home the fact that the statistic had taken up residence in my chart.

Dr. James felt it important that we begin a discussion on the devices available to assist me, stressing that I would not defy the gods of statistical probability forever. Then he indicated that the ultimate decision regarding implanting a device would be mine. I always appreciated being involved in my treatment decisions. Although I consistently took the advice of Dr. James—it had served me well—I still felt like we were a decision-making team. But now I was being told that the ultimate choice would be mine. That was upsetting. It was lonely out on that limb. I wanted him to control the decision, or at a minimum to present me with an iron-clad, logically pure option. The conversation moved on to the merits of an ICD.

Dr. Michael James:

Mike was ready for an ICD. I knew he would be confused. He was back to work, and doing well, handling all the attendant pressures and temptations associated with his job. While he put on weight easily, he was also cognizant of controlling his diet. And he was walking regularly, every morning, even took up jogging because, as he put it, "Walking just became too boring." During his appointments he was alert, cooperative and performing reasonably well on his annual stress tests. In essence, he was feeling good and in control of his life, everything we wanted in a cardiac recovery program.

Understandably, he was puzzled as to why we were talking about "Messin' with a good thing." With Mike I needed to stay ahead of the curve. When he eventually deteriorated, and he would, it would be a quick downhill journey difficult to curtail. The time to take remedial action was now, not when the congestive heart failure and arrhythmias began dominating his quality of life. An ICD was a precautionary measure that would address the arrhythmias before they culminated in a fatal heart attack.

Why an ICD? They work! They save lives! But I wanted Mike to be comfortable with the decision. I carefully explained the benefits and drawbacks of the ICD. In the event of an emergency and the accompanying arrhythmia and low ejection fraction, an ICD would likely shock his heart back into rhythm—and save his life.

We implanted the ICD.

The improvement in mortality following implantation of an ICD is 3% a year, but central to that statistic is that it's 3% every year. For instance, if two groups of 100 were established, 100 with the device, 100 without, at year's end in the group with the devices three more would be alive. Obviously, there is no way to identify ahead of time the three that will benefit, so all 100 qualify. Not the most cost effective way to practice cardiology, but we are improving on that 3% every year.

There are 500,000 pacers, and 500,000 ICDs implanted worldwide each year. Fifty percent of those are implanted in the United States. I'm frequently asked if that means Americans value life more than any other country, or do we gobble up available resources indiscriminately. I hate to think it has to be one or the other.

Electrophsyiologists are kept busy implanting devices. Most of the newer devices have both pacing and defibrillating properties. Although if only pacing is needed, the defibrillating component can be eliminated at considerable cost saving. Mike received one of the newer combined pacing and defibrillating devices. The first time it went off he was in a restaurant. Understandably it scared the hell out of him. The next day we determined the shock was not delivered due to a problem with his heart, rather it was a malfunction of the device. Technically good news; but little consolation to the visibly shaken Mike.

A few years later, however, the device went off several times in one night, literally saving his life. But the downward slide had begun. It was time to discuss other options.

Mike Ranville:

Implanting Dick Cheney's ICD was a tad more memorable than mine.

In layman's terms, after a catheter is inserted in a vein and maneuvered to the heart, ventricular tachycardia (rapid beating of the heart) is induced to test the effectiveness of the ICD. Outside the controlled environment of the operating room, it can be serious.

During the procedure to implant Cheney's ICD, as the protocol dictated, ventricular tachycardia was induced. Dr. Reiner who was in the operating room quickly notified all who were observing that the sudden increase in the Vice President's heartbeat was routine. After the device was implanted, he informed the observers that ventricular tachycardia was going to be induced one more time.

A candid response arrived from the observation deck: "Tell Sung (the surgeon) if he tries to do that again, I'm going to have the secret service shoot him."

For the record, the Secret Service was not present for the insertion of my ICD, and there were no threats of bodily harm when ventricular tachycardia was induced. For that same record, both procedures were deemed a success.

The ICD did not hamper my lifestyle. I adhered to my work schedule—that meant long hours. I continued to play on the same softball team with my buddies. We owned a cottage at the time and I swam and water skied with my daughter, nieces and nephews. Apart from an ever so slight bulge near my shoulder, there was no appreciable change in my appearance.

Early one evening, however, my wife Carol and I were dining at a small restaurant not far from our home. The device went off. I tried to remember what exactly a shock meant and what I was supposed to do. During the ride home I recalled a recent conversation with a few guys who had ICDs. They asked if mine had ever gone off. I said NO, but perhaps a bit too smugly. "When it does," I was told, "you'll remember." Boy, were they right.

First thing next morning—yes it was a sleepless night—I called the ICD clinic. I was told to come in immediately. After lengthy testing, I learned it was the fault of the ICD, not my heart that had generated the shock. I was both relieved and distressed. But what if it went off again? How would I know if it was something serious, or just another malfunction? A frightened and angry ICD patient, separated by only a few hours from a shock, is no one to trifle with.

I dutifully had my ICD checked over the years and the results were both positive and fascinating. Positive because the ICD could, and did, record my every heartbeat since the last check, and could cite the exact time for whatever reason it had begun the journey to register another shock, but then terminated when that shock was deemed unnecessary. Fascinating because it yielded the exact time the aborted journey began. I could go back to my calendar and determine specifically what I was doing that could explain why the ICD was prompted to swing into action. I took great consolation that the ICD stood at the ready to intervene when necessary.

CHAPTER ELEVEN:

Tinker Toys of the Cardiologist

A doctor has a stethoscope up to a man's chest.
The man asks, "Doc, how do I stand up?"
The doctor says, "That's what puzzles me."
—HENNY YOUNGMAN

Dr. Michael James:

Mike tells about one aspect of re-entry into the circle of friends and business associates after his heart attack.

Such is the prevalence of heart disease in society, and such is the dearth of information on heart disease, that he had become, for some, an inadvertent expert on the heart. In the absence of a cardiologist, many friends turned to him for the most basic information regarding cardiac care. After all, hadn't he gone through a harrowing experience and shouldn't he be knowledgeable about the basics, the so-called tinker toys of the cardiologist?

Mike turned his fledgling medical practice over to me, although I believe somewhat reluctantly.

The tinker toys of medicine became available to me as I progressed from student to intern, from resident to fellow, and on to attending physician. When I completed my fellowship, I had at my disposal a thorough

143

and working knowledge of the stethoscope, the chest x-ray, the patient history, the physical and the electrocardiogram (EKG). Collectively they were known as the five-fingered tool kit of the cardiologist. All figure prominently in cardiac care.

They are both familiar and unfamiliar to the general public. While many have heard about them, most have only a rudimentary knowledge of what they actually do and why they are important.

The importance of taking an accurate medical history and conducting a thorough physical are critical components of the diagnosis protocol. I was taught, and after nearly fifty years of practicing medicine, still firmly believe, if you hone your listening skills and pay attention to what patients tell you, you will render a diagnosis that is uncannily accurate.

While the tinker toys, the medical history, and a personal assessment are all valuable, none are meant to be deployed separately in divining a diagnosis. Taken collectively they represent the joining of advancements in the field with medical instinct, both essential ingredients in determining a program of care for the patient.

Further, medical instinct is not derived from operating on a whim. Rather, it is the product of years of schooling and practice devoted to a variety of factors, all designed to provide mastery in caring for the heart. Learning the new procedures and innovations, and how to successfully use them, is an integral part of that training. The program I underwent involved two years of specialized training. Currently, cardiology fellowship consists of three years for the basics and an additional one to two years for Electrophysiology or Interventional Cardiology.

What exactly are the most prominent of those tinker toys?

The Stethoscope

For years, doctors in the movies and on television have dispensed sound advice while adorned with the most basic of medical accoutrements, the stethoscope. Stethoscopes legitimize imparted medical wisdom.

Even today when encountering doctors and physician assistants in a hospital or medical office setting, more often than not they have a stethoscope draped around their neck or jammed into a side pocket of their white coat or uniform.

What exactly is a stethoscope and why does it hold such a prominent position in the arsenal of medical care? What magic resides in that circular piece of metal and concave tubes reaching from the ear that has survived virtually intact, at least in shape, from Normal Rockwell's famous painting, "The Doctor and the Doll" that adorned the March 9, 1929, cover of The Saturday Evening Post? What is learned from placing that stethoscope on the patient's back and chest, then "Gimme a deep breath … Again."

A stethoscope enables a trained cardiologist to recognize the various sounds and noises that signal a valve diseased enough to warrant surgical correction. A heart murmur, for instance, is evidenced by a swishing sound created when the flow of blood through a valve is either too narrow or leaky. While some murmurs are innocent, others indicate a valve that is narrowed or leaky. It's not uncommon to hear a heart murmur in child or young adult that is physiological and innocent. The trained ear can usually discern innocent murmurs from pathological ones. In addition the trained ear can also discern abnormal rhythms such as atrial fibrillation or extra heart beats. Some of these can also be totally benign.

To illustrate, think of a garden hose and turn the spigot so that the stream is narrower, and then listen to the swishing sound. It is the same type of sound heard when listening to the heart, known technically as auscultating the heart.

A positive byproduct of the stethoscope is that when used it allows the doctor to actually touch the patient, an all too rare occurrence in medicine today. I am grateful for being trained in this outmoded diagnostic test, and shake my head at those who do not take the time to properly listen to the heart. When I was in my fellowship, the correction of coronary disease was still in its infancy. Because a vast majority of patients were being treated surgically for valvular disease, it was critical that a cardiologist be trained to recognize the various sounds and murmurs that would indicate a problem.

Mike reminds me that during one of his visits I scolded a Fellow for an inability to correctly listen to the heart, something I rarely do in front of a patient. But proper use of a stethoscope is basic to cardiac care, and, yes, it would exasperate me to encounter a Fellow who had not mastered the use of one of our simplest and yet most effective resources. In recent years my frustration has mounted over the lack of knowledge, or adamantly refusing to learn, how to draw upon this valuable and readily available device. And while it will upset some of my colleagues to say so, many use the stethoscope as nothing more than a piece of medical jewelry. They drape it around their neck and parade around the hospital, but don't know what to listen for—so they never use it.

In evaluating Mike, careful and educated listening gives me a clue as to how hard his heart is working and whether or not his valves are malfunctioning. And it's all being accomplished with the same stethoscope that Norman Rockwell draped around the neck of the wise and kind family physician who adored the 1929 cover of The Saturday Evening Post.

Electrocardiogram (EKG)

"An EKG has been ordered," is a familiar phrase in the lexicon of cardiology. All heart patients get EKGs. And when asking about a friend in the hospital, "What did the EKG show?" seems an insightful and knowledgeable inquiry.

The EKG is a valuable diagnostic mechanism extremely helpful in determining if a heart attack is actually in process, or if one has occurred in the past. It is especially effective when employed for comparing a previous EKG.

Among other things, an EKG can detect a lack of blood flow to the heart, an irregularly beating heart, a heart without sufficient strength to pump adequate amounts of blood to the body, and even impediments that have resided in the heart since birth. Further, the EKG is also helpful in diagnosing chamber enlargement and conduction disorders. It is very valuable indeed.

The usual criteria for diagnosing a heart attack are:

- The typical symptoms: chest pain, pain radiating down the arm, shortness of breath.
- Acute changes on the EKG
- Enzyme elevations (chemical particles that spill into the blood system when cardiac cells are damaged)

A keen suspicion, borne of experience, is also helpful in identifying a heart attack.

Everyone cannot be slotted comfortably into well-established criteria. Many victims have died at home not long after being released from the Emergency Room when typical symptoms were not recognized and the EKG failed to show a typical pattern.

One problem encountered in Emergency Room diagnoses is that when a heart attack is in progress the EKG is dynamic, it changes. But unless there is active ischemia—a shortage of oxygen to the heart muscle—the EKG doesn't change. We needed a test that provides information about reproducible ischemia. One way to combat an unchanging EKG is to perform several EKGs over time in search of typical changes, or "serial EKGs" as it is officially known.

Periodically in the life of a heart patient, EKGs are performed in the office. Comparing the current EKG to the previous gives us a graphic illustration of stability or instability of the heart hiding under the chest cavity. I tell patients after listening to their heart that it's like looking at the hood of a car but now we need to check the engine and the EKG gives us a hint of what may have occurred since the last visit.

Not all heart attacks are recognized by the patient; it is believed that 10 percent are of the silent variety where no discernible symptom occurred. Having said that, I believe a carefully documented history will often reveal a symptom that was ignored or not recognized.

Stress Test

What heart patient is not familiar with the stress test? Although the EKG yields a great deal of useful data, it does have limitations; it is not dynamic. Some patients, when at rest, have severe multi-vessel coronary artery disease and may not have myocardial oxygen supply compromised sufficiently for ischemia—a decreased blood flow to the heart—to show up in an EKG. The other, more obvious, glaring fact is the EKG reflects less than a minute of monitoring the patient's heart rhythm and other dynamic changes. Enter the stress test, and ambulatory monitoring.

The first stress test, or exercise test, involved asking patients to walk up and down two steps of stairs while being monitored by a continuous EKG. We soon discerned certain patterns on the EKG that indicated when the patient's heart was not getting enough oxygen through significantly blocked arteries. The patterns occurred when an artery had at least a 70 percent blockage.

The two steps were soon abandoned in favor of a bicycle or treadmill, both of which are now commonly used today.

The common denominator used in determining a patient's exercise capacity is a Metabolic Equivalent over Time (MET). Age-related heart rate must be achieved in order for the test to be valid. A MET is technically the energy expenditure at rest equivalent to approximately 3.5 ml of 01/min/kg body weight. While few cardiac patients can tell you what a MET is they can tell you how many METs they did during their last stress test.

The most widely used procedure for the stress test is known as the Bruce protocol. It calls for an increase in the speed and grade of the treadmill every three minutes until the patient signals enough. The attending physician can also call a halt to the test because of symptoms, rhythm changes, or certain changes to the EKG reflecting a serious lack of oxygen to the heart.

The information garnered from the stress test becomes valuable when the MET threshold is placed alongside charts that gauge the number of METS necessary to perform various activities the patient seeks to participate in after the heart attack. Stress tests are safe, administered by technicians schooled in exercise physiology as well as CPR. That training is essential to guarding against the patient being in danger while being tested. A cardiologist is also physically in the same area, and monitors the test.

Ambulatory Monitoring

A relatively recent addition to our box of tinker toys is ambulatory monitoring.

Since the EKG gives us less than a minute of cardiac activity, a snapshot in time, ambulatory monitoring or "halter monitoring" as it is known, was designed to allow the monitoring of a patient's heart during an extended period for later playback and analysis. Unlike the ongoing type of monitoring associated with a stay in the hospital where the patient is sedentary at bed rest, ambulatory monitoring enables the gathering of EKG data while the patient is pursuing normal activity. It is done on an outpatient basis. The benefits are valuable: It enables recognition of dangerous rhythm patterns that could be life-threatening, and are preventable. It also allows for the recognition of ischemia during the patient's routine activities that, in turn, enables the setting of guidelines for those routine activities.

To underscore the value of ambulatory monitoring, both medical and fiscal, I recall an incident that occurred while I was at the University of Michigan involving a patient admitted to the Cardiac Care Unit. Ambulatory monitoring was not available. We tried to elicit ischemia or any other arrhythmia, but our efforts proved fruitless due to the patient being at rest. The patient was monitored for about five days. Big surprise—nothing occurred. Given the costs involved in a hospital stay, we termed this the "million dollar EKG."

While an EKG provides an assessment of a moment in time, the heart beats about one hundred thousand times per day, a million times every ten days. Ambulatory monitoring enables an evaluation of each of those heartbeats and data related to discerning patterns critical to the patient's cardiac health.

Information garnered from both stress tests and ambulatory monitoring drive the decisions involved in devising a treatment program for the patient. Further, both procedures are key to determining if a patient is at risk from sudden cardiac death, and what measures are necessary to prevent it.

We frequently monitor the patient for more than 24 hours. When a patient complains of palpitations they are routinely monitored for a month in order to provide adequate time to document the symptoms. We also have implantable devices, such as a computer chip that can be implanted in the office which will monitor the heart rhythm for up to two years. We usually implant this device, called a syncope monitor, in patients that have passed out.

Tinker toys maybe, but all afford indispensable options to the cardiologist.

Nuclear Cardiology

The relatively recent addition of nuclear isotopes to the collection of resources available to the cardiologist represents a major contribution in the diagnosis of ischemic disease, and the ability to effectively follow the patient with documented coronary artery disease. When combined with the exercise stress test, the images give more specificity and sensitivity in the diagnosis and treatment of the cardiac patient with ischemic disease.

It also allows the cardiologist to continually monitor those areas of the heart that cannot be revascularized either with surgery or cardiac stents.

The instrument basic to nuclear is the Anger Gamma Camera, that encodes information on the spatial distribution of a radioisotope onto a two dimensional image. It can identify objects separated by an area as small as one to two centimeters.

Combined with a computer interface, the Gamma Camera can be deployed to acquire electrocardiographically gated images, image based on several cardiac cycles. Computer software then determines right and left ventricular ejection fractions. More importantly, though, it can determine exact areas of the heart not being properly perfused, or supplied with blood and oxygen, during exercise. The advantage of this study is that it is much more sensitive and provides greater specificity when compared to the regular stress test which only monitors the EKG response to exercise. The disadvantage is cost which is close to 8-10 times more expensive. So in patients with documented coronary artery disease whether being treated medically, post heart attack, or post coronary bypass surgery, periodic nuclear testing is part of the annual evaluation.

Echocardiography

After the EKG and chest x-ray, echocardiography is the most frequently used non-invasive test. Its benefits are numerous:

- Echocardiography enables valves to be identified in order to determine if they are too narrow or leaky.
- Echocardiography provides a window to measure the heart chambers regarding their volume and size.
- Echocardiography enables the interventricular septum to be visualized while measuring the fluid around the heart.
- Echocardiography can measure the ejection fraction.
- Chief among the benefits with echocardiography, though, resides in its reproducibility with basically no harm to the patient and no need for IV's or exposure to radiation.
- Stress echocardiography is an alternative to nuclear imaging and yields similar information. Echocardiography watches the heart contract before and after exercise and determines if there is a wall motion abnormality that suggests a lack of oxygen to that area of the heart.

Apart from the benefit it provides, echocardiography represents a fascinating advancement in the field of cardiology and the melding of technology with theory to improve the diagnostic tools available to more accurately assess damage to the heart and treatment programs. It is basically an ultrasound test of the heart, using short bursts of high frequency sound waves that are repeated many times per second producing an image of the heart including the valves and the muscle functions and other sophisticated measurements.

CHAPTER TWELVE:

The Lotions and Potions of the Cardiologist

"If all the prescribed medication in the world were tossed into the ocean, mankind would surely benefit. To their credit, however, the fish would file suit, and they would win."
—Dr. Michael James

Dr. Michael James:

Before replacing any body parts or opening any chest cavities for surgery, every effort is made to address the problem with medication. Credit must be given to the much-maligned drug industry for their efforts in developing pharmaceuticals that significantly improve the lives of patients, and both defray and delay dangerous invasive procedures. More prudent thought, though, needs to be exercised before casually writing prescription, after prescription, after prescription. Like any good thing medication is often abused. Current overuse of pain killers borders on the obscene.

I've always believed if a patient is on more than four drugs they should request a meeting with their doctor to conduct a thorough examination to determine the benefits and drawbacks of each and every pill ingested.

153

If the doctor swats the request aside, or treats it in a cavalier fashion, then it's time to seek another doctor.

I have been known to provide a unique but beneficial service for my new patients. I ask them to bring in all their meds. I then wheel a trashcan in the room and individually assess every prescription. Those that are beneficial are returned to the patient. Those that don't make the cut are tossed into the trashcan. Admittedly, the medical curmudgeon in me is making more frequent and dramatic appearances. But that curmudgeon is making more sense every day.

Having vented, I am the first to admit the effectiveness of many heart-related drugs...but everything in moderation.

Digitalis

Mike developed congestive heart failure and went on digitalis.

Discovered in the 18th century by William Withering, it was known back then as "purple fox glove," a plant that when chewed helped people with "Dropsy[18]," It was eventually refined into digitalis and for an extended period of time, along with diuretics, represented the only drugs available to effectively treat congestive heart failure.

Digitalis has no effect on the normal heart and thus is reserved for the failing heart. It exerts a positive inotropic effect (improved pumping function) which benefits contractility. Additionally, it reduces conduction and has proven effective in slowing the heart rate of patients with atrial fibrillation. Many newer drugs have surpassed the effectiveness of digitalis and it has taken a back seat to the more recent preparations.

Beta-Blockers

Over the years, digitalis has been replaced by other medications—such as beta-blockers, ace inhibitors and aldactone—to improve the function of the heart. Beta-blockers and calcium blockers have supplanted digitalis for slowing the heart rate in patients with atrial fibrillation. Usually taken

---

18   Later called edema, it was labeled "Dropsy" because the water in the patient had *dropped* to the legs.

daily, they warrant special monitoring for signs of toxicity. In patients with kidney problems they may be prescribed for use every other day.

If any group of drugs is responsible for changing and improving the lives of patients with heart disease, it is the beta-blockers. As their name implies, they block beta 1 and beta 2 fibers that innervate the heart. The overall positive impact is found in their ability to improve the supply of oxygen to the heart by decreasing the demands of oxygen.

When stimulated, Beta 1 receptors cause increased heart rate, accelerate conduction and increase contractility. Beta 2 receptors, when stimulated, cause broncho-dilatation and dilatation of peripheral blood vessels. The beta-blockers have dramatically improved the mortality rate of heart attack victims. They have also proven effective in treating among other things, arrhythmias, including atrial fibrillation, atrial flutter, SVT, some PVC's and possibly ventricular tachycardia. Hypertension has also improved following use of beta-blockers. To clarify, I explain it to my patients as exchanging a Cadillac engine for a Volkswagen engine. You will be able to go just as far but will consume less gas (oxygen) in the process. Thus, if there is a heart condition, then there is likelihood that some form of beta-blocker is hovering nearby.

Further, over the years the effectiveness of beta-blockers has been instrumental in changing the treatment of patients with congestive heart failure by decreasing the afterload, the pressure the weakened heart must press against.

The most common beta-blockers are Propranolol, Metoprolol, Carvedilol, Toprol, Lopressor, Atenolol and Nadolol. While effective, they are not without their side effects—asthma, hypoglycemia, lethargy and impotence.

Calcium Channel Blockers

Calcium channel blockers have proven valuable in treating the symptoms of chronic coronary artery disease by lessening the episodes of angina—chest pains that are both uncomfortable and emotionally unnerving. They are also effective agents for treating high blood pressure, and extremely effective in treating coronary artery spasms, although a relatively rare occurrence. Moreover, they help lower the heart rate in patients with tachycardias—a faster than normal heart rate at rest—especially the ventricular rate in patients with atrial fibrillation.

One of the calcium blockers, Diltiazem, usually given intravenously, has proved especially helpful to patients experiencing new onset atrial fibrillation in the Emergency Room. It is frequently responsible for converting patients back to normal rhythm.

In patients being managed medically for coronary artery disease, calcium channel blockers are usually the second tier of drug added to the program when beta-blockers alone do not control symptoms. Unfortunately, there is no data to support or reject an improved mortality rate in patients with coronary artery disease taking calcium channel blockers. Just as there is little quantifiable data relating to patients with an acute myocardial infarction.

The common calcium channel blockers are Diltiazem, Verapamil, Procardia, Amlodipine (Norvasc) and Nifedipine.

Nitrates

We all know heart patients who carry and use nitro tablets, both from television and real life. For most heart patients it is a staple; they are never without their tablets.

Bluntly, they work. Organic nitrates are among the most common medications prescribed by physicians for patients with chest discomfort secondary to coronary heart disease. Since their predominant purpose is to relax the vascular smooth muscle, it makes sense that blood flow around obstructed arteries would be improved when nitrates are administered.

Nitrates can be administered in a variety of ways; the most common, under the tongue or sublingual, is frequently the method of choice during an acute angina attack. Given in this manner, the nitrate is immediately delivered to the circulation through the very extensive vascular bed in the oral cavity. Its popularity resides in the fact that most angina sufferers experience near immediate relief. However, my preference has always been the sublingual spray, which gets into the circulation even more rapidly than under the tongue. Technically, an even shorter route is intravenous, but obviously an IV must be in place for this delivery method to be effective. While long acting nitrates can be given orally, this particular method takes longer to be administered since the drug must be absorbed then metabolized by the liver before it is delivered to circulation. It's effective for chronic management but has little impact bringing relief during an acute episode. Still another method of delivery is achieved by applying a paste to the skin, my least favorite of all. With the exception of the patch form, it is cosmetically unacceptable.

Again, nitrates work. During an acute angina attack or in the midst of a heart attack, nitrates are the cornerstone of treatment. They provide needed symptomatic relief of chest discomfort and they lower the blood pressure. Their effectiveness, however, must be tempered with a need for close monitoring, especially in those patients with hypotension or low blood pressure.

Therefore, the patient presenting with coronary artery disease should likely be on a beta-blocker. If angina occurs despite beta blockers, then a calcium channel blocker, possibly accompanied by a long acting nitroglycerin product, should be used. For a number of years following his heart attack, Mike was on Nitrobid, a long-acting nitroglycerin product.

Sodium Channel Blocker

I conduct an ongoing audit of patient medications. As new drugs become available, and their effectiveness proven, I readily weave them into the heart care regimen. Ranexa is one such drug.

A relatively new drug, Ranexa inhibits late sodium current, reducing sodium-induced overload in myocytes, which in turn acts to decrease ischemia. If the patient has been on appropriate doses of beta-blockers and calcium channel blockers but is still experiencing angina, the physician might want to start using Ranexa rather than the long acting nitrates. I pursued this course of action with Mike and it proved effective. While I favor this approach, it falls into the arena of personal preference and is not substantiated one way or another by scientific proof.

Anti-Arrhythmic Agents

Anti-arrhythmic agents, or as I call them, "cardiac muscle poisons with desirable side effects" have proven useful. Put another way, there is an area of the heart creating a rhythm disturbance and we are smothering the entire myocardium in an attempt to suppress the area causing the arrhythmia. The real problem is the diseased heart; the way to make the arrhythmia recede is to treat the underlying cause, not unlike treating a fever—get to the cause, usually an infection, and the fever will gradually dissipate.

When anti-arrhythmic agents are used they must be carefully monitored for at least six half-lives of the drug, because almost all have a pro arrhythmic effect, i.e., they may cause arrhythmia. Quinidine sulfate is the classic example. Originally, it was the only drug available to treat atrial fibrillation – but could also cause sudden death.

We learned over the years that the anti-arrhythmic agents used to treat life threatening arrhythmias are ineffective. That is why ICDs have become the standard of care for treating life-threatening arrhythmias. Most of the common anti-arrhythmic agents are used to treat atrial arrhythmias such as atrial fibrillation, atrial flutter, and supraventricular tachycardia.

Before we had ICDs, the most effective drug to treat ventricular arrhythmias was Amiodarone. It's a wonderful drug that causes hypo and hyper thyroidism, liver toxicity, pulmonary fibrosis, and also causes deposits in the eyes. In some patients it turns their nose a purple color so they look like a smurf or Uncle Jed over the holidays. Additionally, it lasts in your tissue for over a month before it is completely metabolized. However, for some time it was the only product available. Now who in their right mind would take a drug that has those side effects?

Our group, TCI, was part of a multi-center trial that proved if patients with poor left ventricular function experienced three Premature Ventricular Contractions (PVCs) in a row over a 24-hour period that the risk of sudden cardiac death was significant enough to justify implantation of an ICD.

It was this trial that changed the standard of care from anti-arrhythmic agents to devices, a great testimony to evidence-based medicine.

At day's end the only real arrhythmia we are treating with these agents is atrial fibrillation – and some of the supraventricular tachycardias.

That list of drugs includes – Betapace (Sotalol); Tambocor (Flecanide); Rhythmol (Propafenone); Pacerone (Amiodorone); Tikosyn (Dofetilide); and Norpace (Disopyramide).

Diuretics

Diuretics are known far and wide as "water pills." An apt description as they eliminate excess water from the patient. Understandably, they are used for the symptomatic treatment of patients with congestive heart failure. Technically, sixty to seventy percent of the filtered sodium load is reabsorbed in the proximal tubule of the nephron, twenty percent in the ascending limb of the loop of Henle, and the rest in the distal tubule and collecting duct. In congestive heart failure, the filtered sodium load is decreased.

Diuretics increase urine flow and sodium excretion by acting at various sites along the nephron to interrupt sodium and water reabsorption. Reduction in sodium and water retention results in reduced ventricular preload and improves congestive symptoms. A reduction of ventricular volume at the onset of ejection may also decrease afterload and improve ventricular function. Furthermore, Thiazides and Furosemide may also have direct vasodilating effects. Diuretics are classified by their action of various parts of the kidney. Their site of action may classify diuretics.

Common diuretics are – Lasix (Furosemide); Bumex (Bumetanide); Demadex (Torsemide); Diuril (Chlorthiazide); Esidres (Hydrocholrthiazide); Zaroxlyn (Metolazone); and Aldactone (Spironolactone).

ACE INHIBITORS AND ARBS (Angiotensin II Blockers)

An angiotensin-converting–enzyme (ACE) inhibitor is a group of drugs used primarily to treat hypertension and congestive heart failure. They accomplish this by relaxing blood vessels and decreasing blood volume which in turn lowers blood pressure and diminishes the demand for oxygen from the heart. As the name implies, they inhibit the angiotensin–converting-enzyme, an important component of the renin-angiotensin system. The drugs usually end in RIL: Lisinopril, Zestril, etc.

Angiotensin II receptor antagonists are often used when patients are intolerant of the adverse effects produced by the ACE inhibitors, the most common of those effects being a dry hacky cough. ACE inhibitors do not completely prevent the formation of Angiotensin II, as blockage is dose dependent. Angiotensin II receptor antagonists may be useful because they act to prevent the action of Angiotensin II at the AT1 receptor, leaving AT2 receptor unblocked. Common names of these drugs are Losartan, Cozaar and Benicar to name a few.

In layman's terms both of these agents take lead pipes (the patient's arteries) and make them more like rubber pipes so that the weak heart has less resistance to pump against and does the same for the hypertensive patient lowering the blood pressure closer to goals.

ENTRESTO

Entresto is a recent addition in the treatment of heart failure. It is a combination of an ARB, Losartan and a new agent, Sacubitril. Compared to Enalapril, it reduces the risk of first and subsequent events of heart failure hospitalizations and cardiovascular deaths following heart failure hospitalizations by 20%-24%.

I personally think Entresto is a real game changer and just as we have moved from digitalis and diuretics as first treatment to beta blockers and ace inhibitors, by the time this book is in print I am convinced the standard of care will be beta blockers and Entresto.

CHAPTER THIRTEEN:

"A Period of Stability

Mike Ranville:

On a Sunday night in September, 1984, an elephant decided to take up residence on my chest. I had a heart attack. But forty-three days later I was back to work.

The last week in December and the first week in January are generally void of any significant business in the Michigan Capitol. Legislators are gone. The various state departments are open but functioning at a more languid pace. Only a week before, the atmosphere was frenzied, chaotic. But now Lansing was in its annual cool-down. Christmas parties dominated the landscape.

I worked at Karoub Associates, the oldest and most successful lobbying firm in town. Jim Karoub, founder and owner, appreciated the long hours his employees invested, the time they were away from their families tending to the needs of the business. It was the price we all paid for success. Acknowledging that strain on the family, he frequently charted a year-end trip to a warm weather spot for his employees—and, most importantly, their families as well—Florida and the Caribbean being two of his favorites.

This year Jamaica was our port of call. It was the first time I actually relaxed since late September when I had the heart attack. "No problem, mon." This was Jamaica; no deeds to do, no promises to keep.

We found a local bar, Marguerite's in Montego Bay, that had cable television where we watched the NFL Playoffs. Many of the games were played in frigid weather; loyal fans bundled up to ward off the cold while players blew steamed breath on their hands to keep them flexible. We sat smugly in the warm breezes that drifted through the open walls of Marguerite's. I even had a couple of Red Stripes, the local beer… everything in moderation. We struck up a conversation with the people at the next table. They had pitched their towels next to us on the beach and we had exchanged pleasantries over the past few days, so they weren't total strangers.

He introduced himself as Jerry Burns. As avid followers of the Big Ten we immediately made the connection; this was the Jerry Burns, former head football coach at the University of Iowa, more recently offensive coordinator for the Minnesota Vikings[19].

It was a fantastic trip. Carol and Mara enjoyed themselves. Considering all the medical problems I had visited on the family during the past few months, seeing them having fun was a huge relief to me. Memories of the week are as clear today as they were thirty years ago.

New Year's Eve: Mara is a New Year's baby and we incorporated celebrating her eleventh birthday into the gigantic New Year's Eve party hosted by the hotel. Partner and good friend Gregory Eaton asked her to dance, a fast dance no less. Eleven year-old adrenaline had met its match in Gregory. After a few dances both were sweating. It was officially declared a draw, rematch still pending.

Giveaway Bob: We got to know one of the hucksters from downtown. His uniform of the day was a ragged t-shirt. As we wandered daily by

---

19 After the trip we read in the paper that Jerry Burns had been named head coach of the Vikings. According to the article the announcement was delayed because Burns was somewhere in the Caribbean and could not be reached. We knew where he was: at Marguerite's, watching the playoff games, pounding Red Stripe beer and munching on giant chicken wings. Joe Garcia, a former coach himself, wrote and congratulated him, wishing him success—but not too much success as our Detroit Lions were in the same division as the Vikings. He wrote a nice note back. Marguerite's, by the way, is still there. It appears to be a bit more sophisticated, but it is still there. *"Water the infield with Red Stripe, m'dear. This round is on me."*

his outdoor shop day he announced "The boss is mad at me because I give everything away. He even calls me 'Giveaway Bob.' I'm getting fired tomorrow, so I don't care. Pick out what you want and 'Giveaway Bob' will discount it." Only thing was, it was the same spiel every day. Tomorrow, and the boss firing him, never came. Mara loved "Giveaway Bob" and his theatrics. At the New Year's Eve Party she grabbed me and directed my attention to a young man in a three-piece suit with a gold chain dangling from his vest pocket, flanked by two lovelies. It was "Giveaway Bob."

Ocho Rios: We climbed the falls at Ocho Rios and marveled at the dexterity of the workers as they nimbly danced faultlessly across the slippery rocks taking pictures of the tourists.

Angela's: We survived a harrowing drive up a mountain to have dinner at Angela's, an exquisite Italian Restaurant that featured autographed pictures of Sinatra on the wall, an outstanding meal, and a stunning view overlooking Montego Bay.

The last night there I went out to walk the beach and take in the amazing sunset one more time. Reflecting on the trip, I had laughed more in the past week than I had since September 23rd, aka Elephant Visitation Day. During the walk I put things in perspective.

Only a few months earlier I had a serious heart attack. At the time I didn't know what the future had in store. I had a great job, but didn't know if I could ever work again.

Here I was, though, in Jamaica, enjoying life, enjoying family, enjoying the kibitzing with colleagues and their families, enjoying the "Giveaway Bob" show, enjoying the NFL playoffs with a Minnesota Vikings coach, soon to be *the* Minnesota Vikings coach. I'll bet that elephant who spent an evening on my chest a few months earlier was surprised.

Dr. James was right; a heart attack did not translate into a sedentary life style that was only a way station on the journey to eternal rest. I ran into Jud Heathcote a couple of times at the YMCA where we both used to work out. He remembered me and we wondered if the rest of the guys from rehab were doing as well as we were. We both felt great.

That walk was a nice way to end the week.

Now it was early 1985. Following the hectic lame-duck session during the final weeks of 1984, I was back at work carrying a full load. It felt great. While life in the Capitol is anything but routine, back in Lansing I resumed the regimen I knew before the heart attack. Again, Joe informed me if I needed special assistance I had to speak up. If I didn't, he would assume all is well. I would be held to the same performance standard as the rest of the guys. No excuses—I was expected to do my job.

I appreciated Joe's approach, more than he'll ever know. The last thing I wanted was training wheels. Moreover, if our competition sensed an enfeebled member of the herd—and they would—the wolves would surely carve me out. I would resign before I became a charity case to the firm; pride and dignity would allow for no other course of action.

My partners were great. Despite some genuinely funny gallows humor, I was treated like everyone else; no Hallmark greeting cards awaited me.

The clients who entrusted their legislative program to my firm and me showed genuine concern. It was appreciated. Many had become close friends as well as clients.

But there was an unspoken caveat. Friendships and a history of success meant little when placed alongside results. Jaundiced eyes searched for the slightest hint of weakness. The burden of proof was on me to demonstrate that I could still run with the bulls. My performance was now viewed under the rubric of what have you done for me lately? The cold hard figures of a Profit and Loss statement hold no quarter for heart patients. To paraphrase the old Chinese proverb—success spawns many friends, while failure is passage to the dreaded inconsequential.

The stress of the job I knew so well galloped back into my life. But I dealt with stress before, and I would deal with it now. If I approached my duties expecting the system to cut me some slack, I would fail. If I viewed the world through the eyes of a heart patient, I would fail. In fact, such was the scrutiny, that if I didn't perform better than I did before the heart attack, I would fail.

It was time to move on; I decided to tighten the chin strap. I kept the famous Satchel Paige quote in my desk—"Don't look back, something might be gaining on you." With Mr. Leroy Paige as my mentor and companion, I went back in the game. Physically I was doing well, certainly much better than before the heart attack. I was up early every morning, alternating between walking and running. My weight stayed down. But there was more than just the physical.

The return to work was accompanied by an inventory of my life. I now had a vastly different perspective on my job, family, and the priorities that would govern my remaining days, however many there were. Let me explain.

Regardless of where I worked writing was always a part of my job. And regardless of where I worked someone else took credit for what I wrote.

As a staffer in the Michigan Senate, before joining the Karoub firm, I wrote a number of speeches, and ghosted numerous op-ed pieces for Senators. At the time I didn't mind that someone else was bowing to the applause my words generated; speechwriting was a part of the job I thoroughly enjoyed. Any hint of resentment was quickly tempered when that difficult phrase I wrestled with appeared in the lead graph of an article on the front page of the morning paper—even if it was attributed to someone else. I reminded myself of FDR's directive to his speechwriters shortly after he was inaugurated in 1933—"All staff must have a passion for anonymity." I didn't need an interpreter. The Senator gets the credit. If he[20] doesn't get re-elected, I don't have a job.

While some I wrote for maintained a distant patrician-plebian relationship with staff, others were appreciative and went out of their way to say thank-you. However, two incidents while working in the Senate will never be forgotten. They influenced my decision to set aside time for my own writing career. .

I wrote a speech for a Senator who had been asked to deliver the keynote address at the annual convention of a prestigious trade association. The speech was well-received. I knew the executive director

---

20   At the time I worked in the Michigan Senate, there were no women Senators.

of the association. She called to tell me that the head of their association's Canadian counterpart was going to contact the Senator and ask him to deliver a similar speech to his members when they met in Toronto a few weeks later. She pointed out the invitation to the Senator would also be extended to an aide, presumably the one who had assisted in preparation of the speech. Three days in Toronto. I was thrilled. It turns out the Senator decided the invitation would be offered to someone on his staff with whom he enjoyed a "close relationship". No longer thrilled, I was pissed. Compounding his callous oversight of my efforts, he had a page deliver an assignment—he wouldn't call himself—requesting I rework the earlier speech to ensure a favorable response from the Canadian audience.

Another instance involved a speech I wrote for a Senator on civil rights. You instinctively know when you've done well; nobody has to tell you. In all humility, I was, and still am, as proud of that speech as any I have ever written. Heady stuff for those of us who go about their daily tasks cloaked in FDR's passion for anonymity. Like his colleague, the Senator drew on his stable of paramours for a traveling companion. "Cheaper this way," he explained to me in hushed tones just off the Senate floor. "We only need one room."

In fairness, not all elected officials think with their groin. There were many truly "honorables" in the Senate while I worked there, Mike O'Brien among them.

Senator Michael J. O'Brien, a Detroit Democrat, was one of my favorites. A colorful character, he easily could have just stepped out of a Damon Runyon novel. Before his election to the Senate, Mike O'Brien was a man of broad experience. Not only did he traverse the back alleys of the city of Detroit, but he also knew the elegant dining found in the rotating restaurant that sat atop the Renaissance Center. And he was equally comfortable in both settings.

Senator O'Brien was asked to speak to a group of police officers from southeast Michigan, many of whom were his constituents. A speech to police officers in general and Detroit Police officers in particular, was a home game. I wrote the speech for him; he delivered it beautifully, adding some distinct Runyonesque words and phrases that not only significantly improved the speech but also underscored his time logged on the streets. He had a gift for language I truly envied. After the applause had subsided, he introduced me as the guy who wrote the speech and "the best friend cops had in the Senate." His compliment was remembered years later when police officers sought the services of a lobbying firm to help retain their collective bargaining rights. Class guy—Mike O'Brien.

I left the Michigan Senate staff in 1982, to accept an offer from the firm of Karoub Associates. A new year had begun. Even though I was no longer a staffer, I still received discreet inquiries asking if I "could just flesh out a few thoughts for an upcoming speech." While I still toiled in anonymity, Mr. Karoub recognized the effort and what it meant to the firm, and rewarded me accordingly. The two incidents, though, with the less-than-gracious Senators still weighed heavy. I wanted my own identity.

I was a member of Karoub Associates; that alone bought me instant passage to many doors in the Capitol and state government. I was by no means a super star, rather an offensive lineman, but I was on the letterhead. If I did my job, the entire firm got credit. That was fine. I pride myself on being a team player.

Prior to that, I was a staffer in the Michigan Senate. If my fellow staffers and I performed well, the Democratic caucus we worked for kept control and we retained our jobs.

The heart attack emboldened me. Driven by the proximity of my own mortality, I wanted a record of my own; something more than crafting words attributed to someone else; something more than being a member of a prestigious firm.

I decided to start submitting articles under my name. I got a lot of rejection notices, but a few did get published.

I wrote a story about Bill Gallagher, the photographer who was awarded a Pulitzer Prize for his picture of Adlai Stevenson, or more accurately, for the picture of the hole in Adlai Stevenson's shoe.

I wrote a story about Archie Ellerthorpe, my recently deceased high school football coach. It appeared in a national publication, *The Sporting News*, and was included in the well-read issue preceding Super Bowl week.

I wrote a story about George Romney's ill-fated "Brainwashing" statement delivered on the Lou Gordon Show and acknowledged as the final nail in the coffin of his presidential campaign.

I wrote a lot of stories, and all had the byline "by Michael Ranville."

The writing was rewarding but time consuming. In order to fulfill my responsibility to my clients and colleagues at Karoub Associates, I got up early to write before going to work, frequently at 4:30 a.m. I wrote on weekends. I seriously doubt I would have been so consumed with my own achievements, were it not for the heart attack.

Then I stumbled on the story of a lifetime, "The Case of Lt. Radulovich." I arrived early to a meeting at the Detroit Public Library and had an hour or so to kill and decided to pursue one of my favorite things to do in a library—roaming through the stacks and reading articles in old magazines. I happened on a 1953 issue of Time Magazine and was drawn to an article on Milo Radulovich, a United States Air Force Reserve Lieutenant and University of Michigan Physics student, who was being cashiered out of the military, not for any indiscretion on his part but for the alleged pro-Communist activities of his father and sister. This was the era of McCarthyism and Milo's story epitomized the guilt by association that characterized the Communist witch-hunts of that period. Milo's story took place in Detroit.

"The case," as Milo's family referred to it, was on the front page of the nation's newspaper for 106 days.

I asked Joe Oldenburg, Director of the Detroit Public Library, if he knew anything about the case. He said many of the principle characters were still around, including Milo's family and one of his attorneys, Kenneth Sanborn.

Magazine articles suddenly paled to the notion of writing a book. I became obsessed with the Radulovich story. But a book meant long hours, a total commitment of time and effort. I recalled the words of Professor

David Ling who mentored my Master's Thesis. "Before undertaking any major project," he counseled, "make sure the topic will hold your interest."

I thought long and hard. I was a heart patient. No matter the staying power of the subject matter, could I handle the emotional and physical stress that would surely accompany the effort? My job already exacted inordinate demands on my time; how would I fit writing a book in, and still maintain more than just a passing nod to my health? An adequate amount of sleep, essential to heart patients, would likely become of casualty of the long hours and emotional stress associated with writing a book, especially one laden with a significant amount of pathos.

To my benefit, Dr. James was a strong proponent of heart patients resuming their lives. I was doing that, but I wasn't sure he would approve of the project. I didn't tell him, or anyone else, except for Carol, of my intent to write a book. As far as those around me were concerned, I was just writing another magazine article.

For the greater part of eighteen months, I burned more than my allotted share of midnight oil. Life was a constant flow of adrenalin; the unbelievable stories from the victims of the Communist witch-hunts that flowed during the interviews, uncovering new and wretched aspects of McCarthyism and the Russian bear that hovered over the country in 1953, and the realization that the subject matter was of sufficient import that my book would be adding a new and warranted page to the history of our country.

As the project progressed, the stress increased.

I worked diligently to gain the confidence of Milo and his family. Once I had earned it, and it was determined I could be trusted, they opened their files and their memories to me. While I was grateful, the responsibility was overwhelming. What if I wasn't up to the task?

At first Milo and his family wanted nothing to do with me. A few years earlier he had been burned by a reporter who was doing a "where are they now" article on him. The reporter ordered a bourbon and water that awaited Milo as he sat down for the interview. He instructed the waitress that every time Milo took a sip, she was to bring him a fresh drink. Save for an occasional glass of wine at a festive occasion, Milo was not a drinker. The reporter kept encouraging him to "drink up." Out of courtesy he would lift the glass to his lips, barely tasting the drink. When the article came out, there was a passage that indicated—Radulovich is obviously pained by the events of 1953. While reliving the case during our interview, he consumed six bourbon and waters.

The family believed I was someone who could set the record straight; someone who would finally lay bare the wretched excess of the toll Joe McCarthy and the "ism' forever attached to his name had exacted on innocent people and their families; someone who would vindicate Milo. I came to absolutely adore the family, and that only served to tighten the vise on my anxiety level.

The book consumed me, never really leaving my conscious thoughts. I kept a pad next to the bed to jot down thoughts that were keeping me awake. I'm sure many attending legislative committee meetings assumed I was intently involved in the issue at hand, frantically taking notes on my legal pad. Actually that legal pad had a line drawn down the middle, one side for the issue under consideration by the committee, the other side for ideas on the book that would creep in my mind at the most inopportune time. Of one thing I was certain—I could not fail Milo and I could not fail his family.

I was nearing completion of the book. If I had a week without interruptions I knew I could finish it.

I had never been a big vacation-taker. We had a cottage on a lake that was 90 minutes away. At best I would sometimes take a Friday off during the summer to get a long weekend in at the lake, but never a week at a time. I figured I was due a vacation.

I went to Joe and asked for a week to finish the book. I agreed to be on call if needed, but I would make the necessary arrangements with the clients whose legislative programs I supervised to ensure there would be no missed meetings. He agreed; I had my week.

I finished the book[21]. There were no emergencies with clients.

To affect closure, the book was no runaway best seller but well-received in historical and journalism circles. Among the readers was George Clooney who drew on the book for the first 15 minutes of his acclaimed movie on Edward R. Murrow and Fred Friendly's confrontation with Joe McCarthy, *Good Night and Good Luck*.[22] To my relief, I did not let Milo or his family down. In fact, Milo and his sister Margaret Fishman became celebrities of sorts.

I revisit those days and months following the heart attack at this time to emphasize that heart disease is not a death sentence. If my story can coax just one heart patient off the couch to an active and productive life, it is worth telling.

Life marched on. I was a participant in life, not just an observer watching it go by from an easy chair.

At work, I was not Mike the heart patient, rather Mike the guy who was the butt of many jokes because he couldn't hear (or now that many years have passed, perhaps the guy who chose not to hear. Heh-heh). Mr. Karoub had retired and I was now one of four partners who owned the firm. I was carrying a full client load and participating in all aspects of the firm.

At home I was not Mike the heart patient, rather Mike the guy who takes out the trash. When my mother neared the end of her life and required many difficult decisions on the part of the family, I participated fully in those decisions.

I wound down my participation in the firm and retired around 2005.

As a lobbyist you deal with both political parties. I have many friends who reside at opposite ends of the political spectrum. After I retired I was no longer concerned who I upset with my political leanings. I wrote letters to the editor, and ghosted others for those who wanted to help but didn't quite know how to say it.

---

21   Michael Ranville, To Strike at a King: The Turning Point in the McCarthy Witch-Hunts. (Troy: Momentum Books, 1997).

22   *Good Night and Good Luck* was nominated for six Academy Awards.

CHAPTER FOURTEEN

The Elephant Returns (Or) "The Night They Drove Ol' Mikey Down"

"I tell ya', I don't get no respect. When I had a heart attack, my wife wrote for the ambulance."
—RODNEY DANGERFIELD

In July, 2010, Dick Cheney received a Left Ventricular Assist Device. Not to be outdone, in October, 2013, Mike Ranville received a Left Ventricular Assist Device. Both were suffering from deteriorating congestive heart failure.

ATRIAL FIBRILLATION – RHYTHMN ABLATION

Dr. Michael James:
The heart is an unbelievable piece of sophisticated machinery, an ongoing miracle. Under conditions of normal rhythm, the heart is driven by its electrical system. An impulse begins in the top of the heart and proceeds down three intracardiac tracts to the middle where that impulse

is delayed one-fifth of a second so the bottom of the heart has a chance to fill. The blood is then ejected.

Atrial fibrillation occurs when the heart no longer beats on its own electrical system; top and bottom are not in sync. The top of the heart is going anywhere from three hundred to six hundred times per minute and the bottom is going anywhere from ninety to two hundred times per minute. The rhythm is chaotic and defined as "irregularly irregular." When this occurs there is a decrease of 25 percent in cardiac output.

Generally, the healthy heart with a normal ejection fraction can tolerate atrial fibrillation for a short time. However, patients with a decreased ejection fraction are often pushed into heart failure, compounded by the very real possibility that clots can form in the heart and cause a stroke.

The increased frequency of atrial fibrillation is approaching epidemic proportions. The figures are not encouraging. Currently, 5 to 10 percent of the population in their sixties, 15 to 20 percent in their seventies, and nearly 20 to 25 percent of those in their eighties, will experience some form of atrial fibrillation.

The other important but lesser known tool of the electrophysiologist is ablation, a catheter-based procedure that in essence cauterizes areas where abnormal rhythms have been detected. It has proved successful in addressing problems associated with atrial fibrillation.

We as physicians must make a decision on rate control versus rhythm control. A great percentage of patients can simply take medication to control the heart rate to below one hundred beats per minute and take blood thinners to prevent strokes rather than take very potent and expensive medications to keep their heart in rhythm. These are critical decisions that are made between the physician and patient. Since there is no real change in mortality or morbidity whether or not the patient's heart is in rhythm, the only reason to choose rhythm control is if the patient is very symptomatic when in atrial fibrillation. This is where a critical choice needs to be made since ablation is an option. This is not a procedure to be taken lightly since the catheters need to be passed through the intra-atrial septum. This means that the septum needs to be punctured – a hole must be made so that a catheter can be advanced to the pulmonary vein where the ablation needs to be performed. Remember that the success rate is realistically 50 percent if performed twice; sometimes the procedure can take six to eight hours. The point is the patient should be very symptomatic before agreeing to this procedure.

So in this day and age the Electrophysiologists (cardiac electricians) are busy putting in devices and ablating abnormal rhythms.

Mike Ranville:

Almost thirty years had lapsed since my heart attack in 1984. Save for some changes in lifestyle—diet, alcohol, tobacco, exercise—my life was not at all that different from someone who had never suffered a heart attack. I was active physically and holding down a job that was noteworthy for its stress.

Dr. James always told me when the downhill slide begins, it will be sudden. It was.

There was no other way to put it, I was feeling just plain lousy, constantly tired. More important, though, the slightest hint of exertion triggered breathing difficulties. I began to taper off my attendance at work. In semi-retirement, I wasn't missed, but clients I worked with through the years still sought me out.

I have a writing room on the third floor of our old house. It contains my computer, research materials and also serves as a refuge from the outside world. Problem was I could no longer scamper up the two flights of the stairs required to reach my third floor den. Halfway up one flight, I had to stop and catch my breath. The same with the next set of stairs. By the time I reached the third floor, it was difficult to muster the energy and adrenaline to write. And that deeply concerned me.

Writing is but one passion in my life. Football in general, the Detroit Lions and Michigan State University football in particular, is the other. While I occasionally attend MSU games, my brothers and I have season tickets to the Lions home games. Not only do we share a love of the Lions but also enjoy the time spent together going to and from the games.

We appreciate and share each other's intensity, and thrive on the "nothing is sacred" humor that passes between us.

There is a school of thought that suggests people won't address a pressing medical need until it invades a priority in their private life. My medical condition was taking a toll on the Sunday afternoon visits to Ford Field to watch the Lions. I couldn't walk from our parking space in a ramp adjacent to the stadium without pausing several times to catch my breath. With a great deal of reluctance, I finally submitted to my wife Carol's suggestion to get a wheelchair. But that only addressed the symptom, not the cause.

The wheelchair did produce a humorous moment. Our seats are in the last row of the lower bowl in the stadium—good seats. Just behind us is wheelchair seating. I thought the far corner of that section to be a convenient place to stash my wheelchair. It was out of the way and did not bother those who were sitting there.

At game's end we went to get my wheelchair—it was gone. Brother Marty took off in one direction, brother Jug the other. Both returned empty-wheeled. Marty had a smile on his face. The woman at customer service was aghast—"They took his wheelchair? I swear, they'll take anything these days." I was able to secure a temporary chair from the same customer service representative who, according to Marty, was still shaking her head in shock and disgust.

The lost chair was borrowed from Eaton County Hospice; their name was prominently displayed on the back. I'm sure the impression was left that I was a Hospice resident and more than likely on one of my last outings. The next day the Director of Ford Field Security called and said they found my chair. I drove down to get it and the Director herself met us and profusely apologized.

Writing, football and work were now all significantly curtailed by my reduced physical capacity. More importantly though, the main priority in my life—my family—was also suffering. Sitting in a chair, reading, or dozing, is not the ideal way to participate in the joys of family. The term quality of life had assumed a new and compelling meaning. Dr. James told me more than once that shortness of breath was an early and convincing indicator that something was amiss.

It was during an appointment with Dr. James that I first heard the term "Left Ventricular Assist Device" or LVAD for short. He predicted that within the year, possibly sooner, I would be wearing one. When he explained what it was, and how it functioned, I recalled a recent interview with Vice President Cheney where he told the world about his LVAD. "My heart," he said somewhat incredulous," is actually being pumped by a device attached to the left ventricle of my heart, and that is powered by a battery worn under my shirt." While I shared his incredulity, I had a difficult time grasping the concept.

Up until now my guide to the world of heart problems and cardiac care was Dr. Michael James, and he was an excellent guide. He suggested transferring my primary care to the University of Michigan, indicating it would be to my benefit to "just get into their system." He received his cardiac training at U of M and still knew a number of the cardiologists there. He assured me I would be in good hands.

I did not go gently. Dr. James had served my family and me well. With the understanding he would still be involved in major decisions I agreed to pursue the transfer of my primary care to the world famous University of Michigan Cardiovascular Center.

Getting in was not automatic; Dr. James made the appropriate calls. Further, longtime friend Dr. Joe Schwarz also contacted U of M on my behalf. When he was in the Michigan Senate, Senator Schwarz was known as the patron saint of the University of Michigan. A short time later I received an appointment notice telling me I was scheduled to see Dr. Todd Koelling.

When I arrived for my appointment with Dr. Koelling I met with a number of people, one of whom proceeded to regale me with stories about his motorcycles. I had no idea why until I read the referral letter sent to Dr. Koelling where Dr. James indicated I was a "rider." While he meant "writer" the transcribing typist picked it up as "rider," leaving the impression I was a motorcycle enthusiast.

At the direction of Dr. Koelling I underwent a series of tests. They revealed the top half of my heart was not beating in concert with the lower half, a condition known as atrial fibrillation. I learned that could account for some of the fatigue. I underwent a series of cardio versions, where the heart is literally shocked backed into a synchronized mode. While successful in the short run, cardio version did not hold in its mission to prevent my heart from returning to A-Fib.

The A-Fib continued. In early August, 2013, I entered U of M Hospital to undergo a procedure known as node ablation. Again, in layman's terms, during node ablation a catheter is inserted and threaded to the heart. Once there, a lesion of scar tissue is created to stop the erratic electric signals. It worked, but for only a short period of time. I fell back into A-fib. A second bout with ablation produced similar results. Ablation was not the answer.

During that two week stay in the hospital excess fluid was systematically drained from my body. With able and controlled assistance from diuretics, more than 30 pounds, all excess fluid, was shed. The loss of weight left me weak, but overall I felt better. But the shortness of breath and lack of stamina continued. I could not ascend the stairs or get to my seat in Ford Field without taxing my lungs.

In mid-October, 2013, the ICD Dr. James recommended—the same ICD I eschewed as unnecessary—earned its place in the Mike Ranville Cardiac Care Hall of Fame. On the night of October 19, 2013, my ICD went off two or three times. While the actual number was irrelevant; what will never be forgotten is that each time was marked by a sudden and definitive jolt, not unlike Muhammad Ali landing a punch squarely on my chest. I hadn't had a good night's sleep in some time and I could feel myself falling blissfully into a deep sleep. I fell back on to the bed. Sleep at last. Like Dick Cheney I thought if this is dying, it really isn't all that bad. I wasn't frightened, just relaxed, and very tired.

I could hear Carol calmly calling 911 on the bedroom phone, urging them to hurry. I could hear my daughter Mara in the background saying she would go down and make sure the door was open for the EMT people. For some fortunate reason she happened to be home.

Death, sudden death in my case, had become a part of life. I didn't talk about it with other people but it was always there.

My Dad died suddenly. I often wondered what went through his mind during the last moments. Was he completely aware of his surroundings, as I was? Was he panicked, as I was not? Knowing him, his thoughts were of his family. Mine were.

Carol urged me to stay awake, to keep conscious, and I fought to do so. Evidently I held on because the next thing I remember was the EMT personnel, stretcher in tow, gathered at the bedroom door. They carried me down the stairs. And as we reached the dining room and prepared to go outside I got yet another jolt.

I was cognizant enough of what was happening to realize that each shock, although extremely uncomfortable, represented modern science successfully doing battle with a fatal heart attack.

I heard Carol directing in a rather forceful fashion, "Sparrow [Hospital in Lansing], not Hayes-Green-Beach [Hospital in Charlotte]." I learned later Carol drove a car to the hospital while Mara accompanied me in the ambulance.

Again, there was no panic. I was just very, very tired. And sleepy.

I took note as we left the house and I was being carried down the stairs of the porch that two ambulances had answered the call. I wondered why but was too tired to ask.

I remained at Sparrow until a bed opened up at the University of Michigan Hospital. Once that bed became available, the middle-of-the-night transfer from Lansing to Ann Arbor was accomplished via ambulance.

That stay involved a meeting with Dr. Koelling who, as Dr. James predicted, recommended I receive an LVAD, or Left Ventricular Assist Device. My only heart related procedures to date were minor compared to receiving an LVAD—a few catheterizations, insertion of an ICD and the cardio versions and ablation, none of which required a hospital stay. I erroneously equated receiving a Left Ventricular Assist Device with those other procedures, a few days at most of minor inconvenience. Thirty-seven days later that minor inconvenience still had me in the hospital.

I am fortunate. Throughout my tenure with heart disease accomplished and talented cardiologists provided outstanding care. While I refer to them as the Holy Trinity of my cardiac care, others with a more secular point of view might say, "Ol' Mike hit the trifecta." Either characterization is accurate.

The first, Dr. Michael James, without question is responsible for the productive life I enjoyed following my heart attack thirty years earlier. He was the architect of my return to a normal life, served as my guardian angel through 30 years of medication and procedures, and patiently filled the role of "explainer in chief" regarding what was happening to me at any given juncture during those 30 years. I am the living beneficiary of his professional resolve to remain current in his field. I can never repay him.

The second is Dr. Todd Koelling, my first cardiologist at the University of Michigan. I trusted him initially because he entered my life under the imprimatur of Dr. James. However, he quickly acquired my confidence on his own. While more reserved than Dr. James, he was direct and looked me in the eye. But I was most impressed with his decisiveness. Following a candid discussion in his office weighing the merits of a Left Ventricular Assist Device, he told me I could think about it and come back in a month, but in the interim my condition would not improve and the assessment would not change. Or, he said, a spot was open; I could enter the hospital and do it immediately.

The last few months of the dwindling quality of life rushed to the forefront of the decision making process. To my family I was little more than a vegetable in a chair. I had vivid recall of what surely had to be Muhammad Ali himself meting out several blows on my chest in one night. I loathed the helplessness that forced me to gasp for breath when walking from one room to another. I was unable to negotiate the stairs to my third floor writing den where I hoped many stories still awaited. Following the

Lions and Michigan State University was reduced to locating the right channel on the television.

The quality of my life, or the lack of it, was systematically robbing me of my dignity. I wasn't pulling my weight around the house, couldn't even muster the energy to take out the trash. Even reading, which I loved, put me to sleep. I became what I dreaded most, a sedentary watcher of television.

I looked at Carol. She nodded. I said to Dr. Koelling, "Let's do it."

Dr. Koelling remained the captain of my cardiac team. While other doctors drifted in and out of my life over the next year, my respect for him and his ability never wavered.

It's strange the things that stand out in my long history of cardiac care. While I respected Dr. Koelling's ability, my personal fondness for him was cemented when he volunteered that he was listening to a book on tape regarding the early 19th century visit of Alexis de Tocqueville to America, and his observations on democracy. I recently read a book dealing with the same subject. Later, when Dr. Koelling was performing a right-heart catheterization, we revisited the same subject.

The third member of the trifecta was Dr. Jonathan Haft. With the LVAD surgery, one other physician quickly assumed a prominent role in the growing list of my cardiac caregivers. On October 27, 2013, Dr. Haft successfully performed the surgery that gave me an LVAD. In the days ahead he would dominate my life like no one ever has, even my Sergeant during basic training. While I always maintained the highest regard for him as a doctor, and was profoundly grateful for his extraordinary skills as a heart surgeon, I harbored a great deal of misplaced anger that was directed at him. He was my ticket out of the hospital, but for 37 days he refused to punch that ticket.

I went to the Intensive Care Unit after surgery. My only memories of ICU are an uncomfortable bed and constant noise, both of which kept me from sleeping. I also remember a visit from close friend and former Congressman Dr. Joe Schwarz, a surgeon himself. His presence and assurance that all was normal, even the uncomfortable bed and noise, was comforting. Joe's visit and his friendship meant a lot.

Despite drifting in and out of sleep I was aware of how uncomfortable Carol must be. At least every regular hospital room had one comfortable chair; in ICU there was only one hard, straight-back chair. I urged her to leave, assuring I would be all right, but she didn't.

At last a room became available and I was transferred. Rooms in the cardiovascular portion of the University of Michigan's sprawling hospital complex are private. Thankfully, no roommate.

Once the drowsiness wore off, I began asking about a discharge date which must have given my team of caregivers a bit of a chuckle.

Every day I waited patiently for Dr. Haft and his group of students. They usually arrived between 10:00 a.m. and 11:30 a.m. Certain things stand out regarding Dr. Haft and his rounds. He was always prepared; he didn't have his nose in a computer trying to quickly decipher who I was and why I was here. I could overhear him in the in the hall reviewing my file with the students. Unlike others, Dr. Haft looked at me, not out the window, not at the ceiling, but at me. For those precious few minutes I was the only patient he had. He calmly and convincingly explained my progress, or the lack of it, what he was looking for from me and what I could expect both in the near and distant future. Like Dr. James he didn't slap a coat of varnish on the medical news. But when the good news finally started to appear, that made it all the more believable and memorable. He included my family in the discussion, asked if they understood what he had just said. He entertained our questions with patience and provided thorough answers. And he treated me with dignity.

He was always accompanied by a raft of students. I liked that. It meant he was considered one of the better surgeons and was regarded highly enough to preside over a learning experience for students. To amuse myself, I began referring to them as "Dr. Haft and the Pips." It would have delighted me to no end if, upon their entry into my room, the students did a choreographed dip and took a bow. Given the boredom of life in the hospital, patients have combustible imaginations and are a more than ready audience for a little medical showmanship. Sadly, though, the dip and bow from the Pips never materialized.

There was one memorable moment that occurred on a Sunday afternoon. My brothers had driven down to watch the Lions game with me. We commandeered the Patient Lounge.

I really wasn't expecting him, or any other doctor, to be conducting rounds on a Sunday afternoon. Yet there he was. And he had this beautiful child with him; she looked to be around five or six years old.

I was impressed, first and foremost, that he was even doing rounds on a Sunday afternoon. If there was an emergency, someone capable surely was on duty, or Dr. Haft could quickly be contacted by phone. But he was concerned enough about his patients to take time from his family to check on them.

We have one child, a daughter named Mara. While billboards tout the importance of fathers spending time with their sons, of providing them with a positive role model for being a man, and a host of other aspects of the father-son relationship, there is something special about "Dads and their little girls." When Mara was about the same age as Dr. Haft's daughter, she gave me a gift, a framed picture with several representations of a father depicting special moments with his little girl. The caption read, "Anyone can be a father but it takes someone special to be a daddy." That picture hung prominently in every office I ever inhabited, and now holds a revered spot in my den.

I have fond memories of Mara coming to work with me. And on that day Dr. Haft's little girl came to work with him. I kibitzed a bit with her, and she more than held her own. The young lady had a definite sense of presence. She was surely Dr. Haft's daughter.

There is something special about little girls and their Dads, and Dr. Haft bringing his daughter to work with him spoke volumes to me and did wonders for my morale.

But it wasn't all Kodak moments between Dr. Haft and me. I chafed at being in the hospital. I was walking the halls far more than expected, attacking my physical therapy with a vengeance and cooperating with every aspect of the valuable guidance provided by the occupational therapists. Dr. Haft would not be able to cite "lethargic patient" as an excuse for not discharging me. Dr. Haft's rounds continued to be informative, but predictably migrated to jousting about my release date. I'm sure he grew weary of me; I sure would have.

Then a light at the end of the tunnel flashed. Three outings were scheduled. If I passed them all, going home was elevated from jousting with Dr. Haft to a meaningful discussion of when.

During the first I went down to the cafeteria—technically referred to as "leaving the floor"—to have lunch with an occupational therapist. No wheel chair. No hospital gown; I was dressed in my own clothes and nothing identified me as a patient. I was indistinguishable from the other civilians in the cafeteria—no big deal to most, but of considerable significance to me.

Lunching anonymously in the crowded cafeteria was liberating. The occupational therapist, Kelly, was a personal favorite from the medical team. We talked about her life, her decision to become an occupational therapist, her daughter. For the first time in a long time, it wasn't about me. Such is my memory of the outing that I can still recall Kelly's father was responsible for her becoming an occupational therapist, and that I had the minestrone soup.

The second outing did not go well. Once again Kelly was my lunch partner, but this time her boss accompanied us. Carol joined us as well. We ventured far beyond "off the floor" and went to Zingerman's, a famous restaurant in the Ann Arbor area.

I do not take medication well. If there is a side effect to a pill, it will find me. Throughout my stay in the hospital my regimen of morning pills regularly produced nausea. On the morning of my second outing medication was ordered to combat the problem. The anti-nausea pill left me weak and groggy.

With help of a walker, I barely made it to an awaiting van that whisked us off to Zingerman's. The food was great, but I had no appetite. Carol loved the potato pancakes. Compounding the problem was the lack of a timely response from the LVAD clinic. One purpose of the lunch was to go through the procedures of what action to take in the event of an emergency. We called the LVAD clinic and were put on hold for eight minutes. Kelly was furious.

I fought a valiant fight but the weakness prompted by the change of medication overtook me. I was forced to cut the lunch short and needed help from Kelly getting to the car. When we got back to the hospital I needed a wheel chair to get back to my room. Certain that my loss of energy at lunch would delay my discharge from the hospital, I was embarrassed, angry and despondent.

With blame for my second outing firmly placed on the medication, we proceeded to the third and final outing. This time there was no hospital personnel, just Carol and my sister-in-law Sandy. We could go anywhere. I jokingly asked where the best Coney dog in town could be had. To my surprise I was given directions. "For just this one time,' I was told, "anything goes."

All went well. The Coney dog was beyond delicious. I recall thinking at the time this just might be my last Coney Dog ever. We made the call to the LVAD office simulating an emergency, and the response was crisp and timely.

Finally, after passing the three tests, I was told I was going home. From my standpoint being told I was headed home did not translate into, "Bring the car around; I'll be right there." I heard only what I wanted to hear. From the moment Dr. Haft intoned the near-sacred phrase, "discharge," my mind had already transported me to the greeting that awaited me from Calvin, the gorgeous, ruffled mutt we rescued months earlier…and the keyboard in my den.

I sat on the bed, everything packed, and waited. And waited. And waited.

Given the daily jousting with Dr. Haft that admittedly crossed the line into whining, I halfway expected him to show up with a "Don't let the door hit you on the way out" card. I would not have blamed him one bit. Finally, we were pulling away from the hospital.

Home was beautiful. While still not scampering up to the third floor, it was a much easier trek than when I had last made the journey. I was writing, and reading—two of God's greatest gifts never again to be taken for granted.

All went well. With help from Carol I made the necessary adjustments to a life with batteries. I also began my nightly wrestling match with the cords that plugged into a machine that in turn was plugged into a wall socket. The frustration associated with trying to sleep remains one of my major frustrations to this day. In that battle, the cords held a decisive edge in the scoring.

The ability to manage the batteries and cords was put to the test when, like many other residents of Michigan, we lost power during the bitter cold winter of 2013-14. To many the loss of power is an inconvenience. To an LVAD patient it is a full-fledged emergency. Mara, my resourceful daughter, quickly took two sets of batteries and the charger to the local fire station. She wisely discerned they would have power. They were more than accommodating. But that was a short term solution.

While hotel and motel rooms were nowhere to be had, we were fortunate a close friend worked in a hotel in nearby Battle Creek. We got two rooms, but more importantly, we got electricity in the process.

We weathered the storm in relative comfort. The following morning we learned power was restored. I was fortunate that Carol and Mara were by my side.

Life went on. I was far more productive than the loathsome period before the LVAD had entered my life. Quality of life was gradually restored.

That spring I decided to resume an already lousy golf game. I took up golf shortly after entering retirement. I was never really any good, but did realize some success before the heart problems set in. Now the swing would have to be adjusted to accommodate eight pounds of batteries and wires sticking out everywhere. Despite some outings that were characterized by a creative deployment of profanity, a swing, not the swing returned. Once the batteries were acknowledged, and appropriate adjustments made, the swing did return.

One barometer of my recovery, of knowing that I was adjusting to my new lifestyle, came when I was able to fulfill a speaking request to a journalism class at the University of Michigan. Back when I was sick, Professor, Jim O'Shea, a talented and fascinating guy, had asked me to address his class. I begged off. The strength was just not there. Now, a semester later, he called again, asking if I might be available. I was thrilled and immediately accepted the invitation.

The book I wrote a book a few years earlier dealt with a University of Michigan student, Milo Radulovich, a victim of the McCarthy witch hunts of the 50's. Speaking to the class was exhilarating for a number of reasons.

My best friend Bob Joseph planned a visit to coincide with the appearance in front of Professor O'Shea's class. Not only was it good to see Bob again, but his insights as to what I should stress during the talk were invaluable.

The students knew nothing about my illness or the eight pounds of batteries I tried to conceal. They cared only about what I could offer them regarding the McCarthy era.

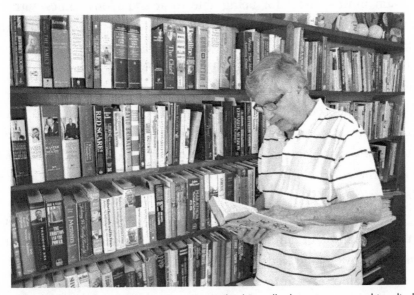

I wasn't Mike Ranville the heart patient. I was Michael Ranville the writer, engaged in a lively give-and-take with some very bright and energetic students. Photo Courtesy of Rod Weaver.

I wasn't Mike Ranville the heart patient. I was Michael Ranville the writer, engaged in a lively give-and-take with some very bright and energetic students. I forgot about the batteries and focused on the issue at hand. Before I knew it the hour had passed. The students applauded. Professor O'Shea was most complimentary, saying I had exceeded his expectations for the class.

In the weeks that followed I received a number of e-mails from the students, all pressing me for greater detail about the Radulovich case and the McCarthy witch hunts.

I was no longer a vegetable to my family, sitting in front of the television. Among other things, the weekly grocery shopping returned as one of my duties, and yes, I take out the trash. Not the most glamorous way to define re-entry into family life, but significant to me. Over the past couple of years I had invoked the "in sickness and in health" clause far too often.

That summer I attended a number of Tiger games. The previous year I went to one, needing to stop several times between the parking lot and our seats. This year I was able to keep pace with my companions.

I am most grateful for being able to attend Lions games with my brothers. The camaraderie and trash-talking between us adds immeasurably to the quality of my life. I was able to ask Dr. James to join us for a game. For the record, he is a knowledgeable football fan and was a great fit when the nothing-is-sacred trash-talking began.

My days are occupied with writing this book. Not only do I hold forth on my care, but Dr. James opines on the state of cardiac care in general, and does not shy from controversy in doing so. We're both hopeful the book will be of benefit to those providing cardiac care, and those receiving it.

I'm also writing another book dealing with famous people I have been fortunate to know, or famous events where I was present. But the point is, I am doing things and leading the kind of life I want.

On behalf of my family and me:

Thank you, Dr. Michael James.

Thank you, Dr. Todd Koelling.

Thank you, Dr. Jonathan Haft.

Regardless of how you came into my life—be it divine intercession and the Holy Trinity of Cardiac Care, or the day ol' Mike hit the cardiac trifecta, your training and your ability have returned my life to me. More than that, you have enabled me to live a life of independence, of dignity. Thank you.

On March 24, 2012, after being on a waiting list for 20 months, Dick Cheney underwent a successful seven hour transplant operation.

All analogies, and parallel paths, eventually die. I was rejected by the heart transplant evaluation panel at the University of Michigan. Dr. James immediately contacted the Richard DeVos Heart & Lung Transplant Program at the Meijer Heart Center at Spectrum Hospital in Grand Rapids, Michigan.

CHAPTER FIFTEEN

"IT'S TIME..."

*"Don't listen to those who say you're taking too big a chance.
Michelangelo would have painted the Sistine Floor, and it would be
rubbed out today."*
—NEIL SIMON

For thirty years Dr. James refused to embroider medical news. Neither of us would be served well if he altered his approach now. He defied the F. Scott Fitzgerald admonition that "there are no second acts in American lives" and delivered an impressive rewrite of the second act of my life. But I am well into the third and final act, closer to ringing the curtain down than raising it.

The LVAD was a success, no question about it. It did exactly what it was supposed to do. However cumbersome the batteries during the day, and however confining the wires at night, I still fared much better than during the pre-LVAD days.

Significant to me, I was able to read and write again. Both were severely curtailed in the days leading up to receiving the LVAD. An inability to concentrate rendered both reading and writing virtually impossible. Moreover, a lack of energy significantly suppressed any desire to do either. My writing room is on the third floor of our old house; the energy required to negotiate three flights of stairs was just not there.

The LVAD changed all that. Unlike before, a book in my hands didn't automatically trigger a nap. And while I wasn't exactly scampering up those wretched stairs, I was at least navigating them. And I reunited with my old and dear friend the keyboard.

A difficult decision confronted me, namely, should I pursue a heart transplant?

Life with the LVAD certainly had its challenges. But I was once again alert, and enjoying the things most important to me; family, reading and writing, and sports. When compared with the pre-LVAD days, life was infinitely better. The wires and batteries were annoying, sometimes reaching the point of anger, but as was pointed out to me by Dr. James, "Consider the alternative." Now with a heart transplant entering the discussion, the definition of "alternative" had broadened, some would say considerably, and not all of it was positive.

Was I foolish in risking the good to pursue the great, with the great being hazy at best? The LVAD had rescued me from lethargy and daytime television; the dramatic change it brought to the quality of my life could not easily be dismissed.

The transplant surgery was complicated and fraught with significant risk, an all-out assault on my body and mind. And that's assuming I even survived the surgery. While ninety percent live to tell the tale of their transplant, ten percent do not. Would I become one of those who made the top half of the class possible?

Was my pursuit of the ill-defined and elusive great fair to my family? Had the "in sickness and in health" clause had been invoked for too often in recent years. Was I asking too much, especially given that the status quo was tenable?

How would I react? Would a new heart add life to the additional years it promised, or would something go wrong causing me to revert to the dismal existence of the pre-LVAD days? I was told time and again, "There are no promises."

I am aware that life expectancy for an LVAD patient is at best six to eight years, the life of a transplant recipient ten to twelve years. Despite the vital function an LVAD presents, waging a daily battle with the batteries and wires was a constant source of frustration, never reaching the point of routine. And while the decision to provide a new heart cannot be driven by convenience, I told all who will listen, unlike some recipients, the additional years conferred on me by a transplant will not be spent in front of a television or invoked as a ready excuse to resume smoking. Only those too shallow to comprehend the significance of this cardiac miracle—the transfer of a pulsating heart from one body to another—would spend the additional years awarded them in lethargic pursuit of another day of television watching. Failure to embrace the additional years as an incredible opportunity to make a contribution is to visit disrespect on both the donor and the donor's family.

After a great deal of thought I decided to press my cardiology team at the University of Michigan to begin a discussion on a heart transplant. In response, I was ushered through a number of tests intended to evaluate all aspects of my health. The tests were designed to ensure I did not receive a new heart and then have one or more other organs in my body fail. The results of those tests indicated the condition of my other organs would not be a negative factor in securing a new heart.

My spirits were buoyed when I was asked to meet with the transplant administrator. If the march down the bureaucratic trail had begun, I reasoned U of M must be serious. The meeting went well and I was even asked to sign papers indicating I would not use alcohol or tobacco products. So specific were the boundaries of behavior that I was warned to stay out of casinos as the second-hand smoke could trigger a tobacco alarm. Neither restriction was a problem.

I waited anxiously for the evaluation committee to convene on my case. Coming from the political arena, I instinctively wanted to know who served on the committee. Would it be possible to visit them individually to plead my case one-on-one? So many times during my career a course of action had been predicated on a "vote count." Now that vote count took on far greater import than any bill moving out of committee.

I was told the process is carefully structured to prevent outside interests from influencing the decision, and that any attempt to do so might work to my detriment. While I abided by the counsel to stand clear of those rendering the decision, frankly the admonition smacked of hypocrisy, perhaps not as it specifically pertained to the University of Michigan process, but certainly to the overall paradigm that governs the harvesting and awarding of organs.

As a baseball fan I was keenly aware of the controversy surrounding Mickey Mantle's abbreviated stay on the list for a liver transplant. LifeSource, the organization that presides over organ and tissue donation, vehemently denied Mantle received preferential treatment. However, he was transplanted after spending only one day on the waiting list. He died two months later of liver cancer. Considering the well-publicized lifestyle that likely contributed to Mantle's health problems, serious questions surround the decision. Res ipsa loquitur," the facts speak for themselves." Could, or should, the liver have gone to a recipient who had logged fewer hours on a bar stool? Additionally, at the time of Mantle's death in 1995, transplantation for patients with liver cancer was not a proven approach; yet he was transplanted. LifeSource responded with a statement indicating the decision to transplant Mantle was driven by the fact that he was only days, perhaps hours, from death.

Despite assurances to the contrary, my concern that the process could be gamed, endured.

Steve Jobs, the highly visible CEO of Apple Computers, received a new liver following his listing at multiple transplant centers. Ultimately he received a transplant in Tennessee where the wait was much briefer, not in California where he officially resided.

The committee, Dr. Koelling informed me, voted to reject my request for placement on the heart transplant list. Further, the decision would not be revisited, not now or in the future.

My candid conversation with Dr. Koelling, the cardiologist who held superintending authority over my care at the University of Michigan, indicated I was rejected due to the fact that my health likely would not deteriorate to the point of requiring a heart transplant for another three to four years, presumably around age seventy-three or seventy-four. At that time I would be too old.

The news was devastating. I was bitter, and I felt used.

Prior to learning of my rejection I was asked to tell my LVAD story to a number of prestigious groups. One occasion involved a dinner for the University of Michigan cardiology community at the tony Dearborn Inn. I assumed the podium following a power-point presentation that included some sobering statistics. LVAD patients last between six to eight years; I was approaching two years with mine.

My opening comment: "It's a bit disconcerting to see your mortality bandied about and then reduced to a point of intersection on a graph in a power-point presentation" – was a toned-down version of what I really wanted to say. I was angry. As I was handed the microphone, the legendary gladiator greeting to those who had gathered in the coliseum to be entertained by the death of one of the combatants rushed to the forefront of my thoughts: "We who are about to die salute you."

Before speaking I had to pause in order to compose myself. I needed a moment to separate myself from what I deemed a callous disregard for how I would personally accept the fact that the previous presenter had just assigned me a termination date, and one in the not too distant future.

Apart from the transplant committee's decision to not place me on the list, my reaction to the presentations that evening represented the only blemish on an otherwise great experience with the University of Michigan cardiovascular team.

In retrospect, I should have realized the audience before me and grown a few calluses. While devoted to healing, that audience regularly confronts death. Examining death with cold and calculating eyes is necessary when fashioning greater measures for healing. Still, it took me some time to overlook what I deemed was an after-dinner program that treated my remaining days in a cavalier manner.

Weeks before at a gathering of medical students I was asked outright my feelings about death, namely my death, and the fact that it had inched closer, to a point that it was now in sight. I decided to take the lighthearted route and responded with a Woody Allen quote: "I'm not afraid of dying; I just don't want to be there when it happens."

The committee's rejection of my petition to transplant crippled me emotionally. There were many things still to be done before a priest chanted over my casket.

I turned to Dr. James, the one guy in a white coat with a clipboard that I unequivocally trusted; the one guy I knew who wasn't reluctant to fight for his patients and challenge a bureaucratic guideline that warranted additional scrutiny; the one guy whose medical acumen was responsible for adding life to the thirty years that had passed since the onset of my heart problems; the one the one guy I knew who would not "pee on my shoes and tell me it's raining."

Dr. James immediately began a discussion that involved a heart transplant from another institution—Spectrum Health, in Grand Rapids. After a review of my records and recent tests, I was accepted by Spectrum Health and placed on the waiting list for a heart transplant. All of my cardiac care was transferred to Spectrum Health.

There was no dip in the quality of care following the transfer from the University of Michigan to Spectrum Health. That made it easy to debunk those who asked, "Aren't you concerned about leaving the world-famous University of Michigan Cardiovascular Center?" While I am grateful to the medical team at U of M who cared for me, the answer is NO! My confidence in Spectrum Health is justified and unfailing.

Still shattered and dismayed by the rejection from the University of Michigan, especially given the positive feedback my presentations generated, I replayed in my mind Dr. Koelling's call informing me I was not eligible for a transplant. I wanted to throw down the red flag and challenge the ruling on the field.

What unknown variable hovered over the committee's deliberations? The competitor in me wanted the opportunity to refute the finding, but first I had to know what drove the decision. Dylan Thomas and his admonition, "Do not go gently into that good night," aptly described my frustration. "Rage, rage," Thomas urged, "against the dying of the light." And I desperately wanted the opportunity to do so. After years of brawling in the back alleys of the political arena, I instinctively knew "It's not the earth the meek inherit, it's the dirt.[23]"

I passed all the physical examinations; should a new heart become available it would not be placed in a body with failing organs.

The counsel of good friend and golfing partner Kurt Chubner proved valuable. The conversation between holes was frequently devoted to heart disease in general and my potential transplant in particular. His blunt message:

"Frustration will be part of the success equation. Results will occasionally fall short of expectations. You are a goal-oriented person with a strong discipline to achieve success. After all, I've seen you on the golf course, beating your fairway wood repeatedly on the turf after an occasional errant shot gone astray. There can be no more kicking the dog as a stress release mechanism on exercise days that fall short of improvement. You owe the donor and the donor's family respect. You owe them a more active life than just sitting beside a phone waiting for a call. You owe them a healthy lifestyle. You owe them a productive life. Anything else would be dishonorable."

Kurt is not a coddler.

I obsessed regarding what I could have done differently.

Once the smoke had cleared, however, Dr. Koelling's final statement could not be massaged or misinterpreted, "The committee's decision is final and will not be revisited."

The Call

While I was consumed with frustration at U of M's rejection, grass was denied life under the feet of Dr. James. On the same day he learned of the decision at U of M, he contacted Dr. Michael Dickinson, Heart Transplant Medical Director at Spectrum Health. With Dr. James in the

---

23   A line from *Camelot*, lyrics by Allan Jay Lerner, music by Frederick Loewe.

lead, a case was mounted for consideration of a heart transplant. I was placed in the second tier, deserving but death not imminent. Spectrum Health, to my benefit, accepted the results of the preliminary tests ordered at U of M.

The next few weeks were devoted to meeting with the extremely capable transplant team at Spectrum.

The surgery, as I was already aware, was complicated. Recovery was lengthy and difficult, both for the patient and family. There were side effects to the lengthy list of medications, some could be quite unpleasant. I could incur some loss of motor skills.

There was also a sobering conversation regarding risks that accompanied the surgery. Ten percent die on the operating table. It's difficult to tell yourself to relax, that you automatically fall into the ninetieth percentile. That 10 percent figure had to be derived from somewhere. Another 10 percent do not survive the first year.

Periodically Spectrum Health scheduled appointments to ensure I was still a viable candidate, both physically and emotionally. The close monitoring enabled an assessment to determine if my physical condition had changed to a point where I would be disqualified, or to ascertain if I was having second thoughts regarding a process that no matter how many times it is performed is anything but routine. I learned the precise attention to detail that characterized these sessions was geared to ensure that when a heart became available, the process could move with needed dispatch and not be hampered by a failure to satisfy a bureaucratic concern that should have been addressed earlier.

With each visit I inched closer to meeting the surgeons, Dr. Martin Strueber, and Dr. Asghar Khaghani, one of whom would be wielding the scalpel for my transplant.

During the assessment meetings Dr. Strueber dropped in more than once. He had an impish, all-knowing half grin that translated into confidence without arrogance. His demeanor was calming. I felt comfortable with his hand at the till during the surgery.

On August 28, 2015, my mind was focused on golf. Occasionally, good friend Pat Murphy and I stepped out on the links. Pat and I graduated from the same high school, Flint St. Agnes. A three-sport star, he was one of the better athletes to have ever attended St. Agnes.

I won the first match played earlier in the summer; Pat won the second. Decorum and good sportsmanship had given way to trash talking that had long since abandoned all pretense of civility. A political reporter by trade, Pat's command of the language more than armed him for our verbal jousting. I was eagerly anticipating the grudge match with Murph.

We were just approaching the first tee when my cell phone rang. It was Carol. "You'd better come home. Spectrum just called." I told Pat. He wished me well. Later, he would discard all sense of Christian charity acquired at St. Agnes and claim victory in the best of three series, maintaining transplant or not, I had just forfeited the final session. I assumed at one point in his career he interned in the Nixon White House under Charles Colson.

I rushed home. Carol drove to Grand Rapids. Anxiety was having its way with me; I was in no condition to drive. The 10 percent casualty rate, not the ninety percent survival rate, was consuming me.

My mind was racing. I wondered who would come to my funeral. Would anyone ask to be heard and say something nice about me? For some time, Carol had been urging me to control the moment and write my own obituary. Now I wished I hadn't put it off.

What if the whole after-life thing was nothing more than a ruse and death equated to true finality? Conversely, would I be able to see friends and family, play football and baseball again? I pondered the question everyone wanted the answer to, but nobody until Mark Twain had the courage to ask—is there sex in the afterlife?

Those were my last conscious thoughts until I woke with a raging thirst trying desperately but unsuccessfully to talk. My mouth wouldn't engage. Carol and Mara said I quipped that I sounded like Kirk Douglas after his stroke. That made them both laugh and relieved concerns of brain damage stemming from the surgery and five days of induced sleep[24]. As a result, I lost total track of time; I was completely disoriented—understandably so. During that time fluids were pumped into me causing my legs to swell beyond recognition. I had "elephant legs."

After doing battle with the cobwebs that had invaded what remained of my thought process, I learned a transplant had taken place, and it was successful. I couldn't make the connection between my grogginess and a transplant—what transplant?

I remember being relieved that I was awake. I had wild dreams. While struggling for lucidity I was aware enough to realize that the effort to acquire some control of my immediate surroundings meant I was free of the dreams. One dream in particular I remember to this day. I had offended someone close to my good friend Joe Schwarz. How or why I didn't know, but I was desperate to talk to Joe and apologize.

The room slowly acquired definition and clarity; I became more alert. The first faces I saw were those of Carol and Mara, both smiling, both assuring me that all went well with the surgery. Seeing them aided significantly in re-ordering myself to the present and that I was in a hospital. Even the remote notion of a heart transplant was starting to make sense.

Carol buoyantly announced, "You got a new heart, Mike!"

I think my response was an erudite, "Oh yeah?"

I was parched. Knowing that patients in a hospital usually had a jug of ice water at their bedside, I asked for a drink of water, but was told the doctors said I couldn't have any. I calculated the no water directive was issued by Dr. Strueber. So great was the thirst that his perfect ten approval rating was in jeopardy. I was offered a few ice chips, emphasis on a few. The uncontrollable thirst would never leave me for the duration of my thirty-day stay in the hospital. I actually dreamt about a glass of cold water.

---

24   I doubt even the great Henny Youngman ever got a laugh only moments removed from five days of induced sleep.

I was moved to the Intensive Care floor. My stay there did not go well. I regularly fought with the nurses. My attitude was atrocious. I'm sure the nurses were claiming in unison, "Taking care of jerks like him is not why I went to nursing school."

There are reasons for my appalling behavior, not that it matters now as the damage has been done. Looking back, I applaud those nurses who surely must have labored in anger. They did not allow the excellent care I received to be influenced by my horrendous attitude. I would like to take a moment for a personal privilege and provide my view of the world at that time.

I was thirsty, the depth of which I had never known. Occasionally a nurse would give me a few ice chips, but only a few, and only occasionally. While the ice chips helped, they were a sorry substitute for water.

I am not a difficult person by nature. Laughter is a frequent guest in my interaction with people. But I had been reduced to begging for a few lousy ice chips. I felt that was an attack on my dignity; it greatly increased my level of agitation. I did not suffer in silence, lashing out at whoever was closest to the glass of ice chips. They started charting my ingestion of chips.

"Could you give me a few ice chips, please?"

"I'm sorry, but you just had some. You still have to wait eighteen minutes for your next spoonful."

"In eighteen minutes there won't be anyone around."

"You're not the only patient on the floor."

"And you're no Mother Theresa. Look, I'll sign a paper absolving you of any legal liability resulting from an ice chip overdose."

"I don't make the rules."

"But you sure do delight in enforcing them, especially if it increases my discomfort. I don't know what the hell is going on, but a few lousy ice chips are not going to alter the natural order of things."

"Your complaining does not help your cause. I'll see you I eighteen minutes."

The frustration mounted.

I am claustrophobic. Most non-claustrophobics think the malady is confined to an aversion of close spaces. There's more, and it made my stay total misery.

The same bed. The same four walls. An unrelenting 24-7.

The bed is uncomfortable to begin with. I only wanted to shift my position and dangle my feet over the edge just to restore some feeling in my back and legs, to break the oppressive monotony that dominated those sterile walls. Any disengagement from the bed or the hospital version of an easy chair, no matter how slight, set of all sorts of alarms. The alarms triggered the appearance of an armada of medical personnel, no doubt the hospital version of DEFCON 4. Upon seeing me sitting on the edge of the bed, feet dangling, the scolding began. The errant child is at it again.

The errant child is extremely anxious. The bed he is confined to is small. Just knowing that breaking the plain of that bed will summon the SWAT team produces the same discomfort that would be generated by an enclosed space. The parameters of the bed become the new enclosed space. And just knowing that my world began and ended with the bed's four corners exacerbated an already high level of stress.

No one took the time to ask why I was agitated, why I seemed to have a blatant disregard for hospital rules, why my chest was heaving while being escorted back to that small, confining space.

"You have to rest," said the out-of-patience nurse. I would have loved to rest. In fact, I was exhausted, but rest is impossible when your mind is galloping with the emotional pain and discomfort that afflicts claustrophobics, at least this one.

When confinement is paired with a thirst that has been raging for days, the outgrowth can, and was, highly combustible. The new heart had to be saying, "This guy has got problems. I'm not going to last long here. How do I transfer out of this outfit?"

My deportment problem has another contributing factor that is squarely rooted in dignity.

When a young lady, in this case a nurse, refers to me as "honey" or "sweetie" it is not flattering, it is demeaning. Assuming you're giving this old dude a thrill by employing a term of endearment is condescension at its worst. The problem is far worse in restaurants.

My distorted sense of reality translated the comment as, "Poor guy. More than likely no one has flirted with him in years. Think I'll give him a cheap thrill and call him 'sweetie'."

Had my discomfort reached the point where I resented an overture of kindness?

Thirst + claustrophobia + being treated in a demeaning fashion = an agitated patient.

My behavior had consequences far beyond the parameters of my bed and the sterility of four walls. I was making life miserable for Carol and Mara. My personal comfort and myopic view of the world took precedence over all, even the two people I love most on this earth. I will carry my regrets for the pain I caused them to my grave.

The calls, cards, and letters from family and friends always seem to arrive at a time when morale was low. And they always provided a sorely needed boost. In that regard, visits from extended family also brightened the day.

Visits from Dr. Joe Schwarz were not only welcome but informative. A practicing surgeon, Dr. Schwarz was most helpful in allaying fears generated by the surgery and the discomfort that accompanied it.

The visits by Dr. James, who was logging his thirty-second year as my cardiologist, brought more comfort and reassurance that all had gone well than any anti-anxiety pill. Not only is he an excellent cardiologist and writing partner, but also a good and loyal friend.

SPECTRUM HEALTH

On August 28, 2015, I received a heart transplant in the Richard DeVos Heart & Lung Transplant Program at the Meijer Heart Center at Spectrum Hospital in Grand Rapids, Michigan. I had no idea of the culture, history and tentative starts that preceded my surgery that evening.

More than twenty years earlier discussions began in earnest regarding the direction Spectrum Health (then Butterworth Hospital) should take with regard to cardiac care and particularly heart transplant. While they wanted to pursue it, the time ran out on a Certificate of Need they were granted and the issue was put aside. An authorization from government designed to control the proliferation of health care facilities in order to control costs, a Certificate of Need, is, by design, difficult to acquire and includes a termination date.

Local leaders dreamed of someday being able to provide for all the medical needs of West Michigan in their community. This vision drove the merger of the two hospitals with open heart programs (Blodgett and Butterworth) to create Spectrum Health and was the launch of the "medical mile" in Grand Rapids, a multi-billion dollar investment by the Van Andel Institute of medical facilities along Michigan Avenue.

Thus in 2004, two open heart programs became one, and Spectrum Health rose to be among the leaders in the volume of cardiovascular services performed in the state of Michigan. Those services included open heart surgeries, stents, heart catheterizations, electrical ablations, and echocardiograms. But noticeably absent was the next generation of cardiac care, Left Ventricular Assist Devices (LVAD) and heart transplants. They asked themselves, what's next?

Spectrum Health hired a consultant to do a feasibility assessment to provide options and directions to chart the path that could or should be traveled. The results fell woefully short of what they sought. The study said you could – or you couldn't. It didn't really help and it didn't give them the answers they were seeking.

According to Dr. Michael Dickinson, Heart Transplant Medical Director at Spectrum Health, "We should have examined ourselves." As an initial step they decided to pursue offering LVAD only.

At the time if a patient was offered an LVAD or transplant it was dependent on the local physician's knowledge and willingness to pursue advanced therapies. Many of those physicians had not seen or were not familiar with the therapies; they were not part of their retinue of cardiac services. Transplant and LVAD was still unique.

"Heart failure patients die within five years," Dr. Dickinson explains. "For a physician, medicine helps. But essentially they were only managing decline and death. If, however, the physician was familiar with LVAD and transplant therapies, both became a viable alternative."

Geography played a factor. In 2007, if a heart failure patient was a candidate for an LVAD or a transplant they likely resided in Southeast Michigan. The rest of the state was severely underserved. Patients living near a transplant or LVAD center were two-thirds more likely to be offered a transplant than those not living near such a center.

In 2009, Spectrum Health performed its first implantation of a Left Ventricular Assist Device. Before embarking on offering LVADs, and later transplants, Spectrum Health was sending the majority of their patients to Northwestern Memorial Hospital in Evanston, Illinois. While the medical care was superb, it came at a tremendous inconvenience to patients and their families. Not only was Evanston a day's drive from Grand Rapids, parking at Northwestern was thirty-six dollars a day.

After many meetings in nearby Chicago, Spectrum Health decided to pattern their cardiovascular program after Northwestern's, and other Chicago-based programs, sans the thirty-six dollars a day parking. In that regard, Spectrum Health reasoned their patients would fare better if they didn't have to worry about families being inconvenienced during their stay in the hospital. They had already erected a hotel in close proximity to the hospital where families could stay at minimal cost[25].

The first step, not an easy one, was to secure a Certificate of Need from the State of Michigan. One provision of that valued credential specified that a successful heart transplant be performed within eighteen months, the same provision that prevented them from performing heart transplants years earlier.

The task was formidable, but this time they determined success was the only option.

---

25   I am but one of many grateful patients for that service.

They needed to recruit a qualified transplant surgeon, build the program, evaluate patients, get the patients listed, and then wait in line for suitable donor organs. At the time, the average wait from listing to transplant in the state of Michigan for a heart transplant was 13 months. If the timeline was accurate, it would leave only five months to completely fashion a new transplant program, including recruiting and hiring a transplant surgeon.

The brief history is worth noting, if for no other reason than it is a story of determination and conviction.

Butterworth Hospital was granted a certificate of need to do heart transplants. They went about recruiting a surgeon but he arrived only weeks before the 18 month window closed. There was not enough time to start a program and the idea of heart transplant went quiet for a number of years.

In the interim, a group of regional leaders boldly dreamed of creating a medical powerhouse center in Grand Rapids. They determined if the two larger hospitals merged into one, it would create an exceptional medical facility large enough to provide not just the usual care, but also enable assumption of the advanced care that patients currently received only after traveling to Ann Arbor, Detroit, Cleveland or Chicago.

The journey from dream to reality was challenging. The Federal Trade Commission objected to the merger. Ultimately, after assurances of a not for profit entity with commitments to the community good, the merger was approved. Coincident with the merger was a great philanthropic effort to build a physical plant up and down the hill around Butterworth Hospital. It became known as "The Medical Mile" and included beautiful state of the art buildings, and "The Meijer Heart Center," a new heart hospital named after the key philanthropist who helped make it possible.

With the opening of the Meijer Heart Center the question of heart transplant could be considered again. In 2007, a group of physicians and leaders at Spectrum Health began to explore the feasibility. By 2008 they decided to pursue a ventricular assist device program without transplant, but in 2009 a window opened to challenge the state standards around heart transplant. With this, came approval of the critical Certificate of Need for transplant at Spectrum Health. On February, 19, 2010, Spectrum Health was given the charge to begin performing heart transplants within 18 months.

In September 2010, Dr. Asghar Khaghani moved from England to Grand Rapids and become the transplant surgical director, with Dr. Michael Dickinson appointed to serve as the transplant medical director. The program and teams were assembled and by November 1, 2010, the first patients were put on the transplant waiting list. On November 27, 2010, a donor heart became available and Dr. Asghar Khaghani performed Spectrum Health's first heart transplant.

Many other notable cardiac landmarks dotted the way. And, of significance to me, in 2014 Dr. Martin Struber, internationally renowned cardiac surgeon, was recruited to join the Spectrum Health team. The following year he presided over my transplant.

***

I grew up loving the show tunes from old Broadway musicals. I'm sure it stems from my mother's ability to play any song that waltzed into her mind. The vast majority of the melodies that came out of that old piano in the living room were from Broadway. Our house was filled with music. Mom was really good.

In college I had to fill an elective requirement. With Mom's show tunes lurking in the wings, I decided to take a course in theater production. The syllabus indicated all students were required to work on an actual production. I chose a show that was essentially a Broadway montage; lots of Mom's show tunes, and, for us grunts taking the course as an elective, lots of set changes.

While Mom gave me a love of Broadway music, God did not cooperate by providing me with a Broadway voice. I became a crew member, those unheralded souls responsible for the invisible rush of activity that occurs when the stage darkens and two minutes later those blessed with the

Broadway voices hold forth in a brand new setting. We took no curtain calls but did take consolation in the knowledge that without us the show would not have gone on.

I cite that class now because the crisp organization and precision that governed the production left a telling mark on me. While mine were only minor tasks—putting a table next to an easy chair, for instance—the next number would not have worked if that table wasn't there. We all had jobs, and the success of the production relied on us doing those jobs. It worked liked a fine Swiss watch. No small roles, only small actors.

Memories of that class surfaced after the initial meetings with the Spectrum Health heart transplant team. While it is not my intent to equate the complexity and import of a heart transplant to a college production of Broadway tunes, the comparisons helped me sort out in my own mind the carefully crafted process I was encountering.

Crisp and precise accurately described the system at Spectrum Health that readied me for my transplant and the follow-up care. Carol and I met a number of the team; all were friendly, but all were professional. No question lingered in want of an answer. The confidence that governed the discharge of duties brought a sense of comfort to this anxious patient and his family.

My observations, I learned later, were wholly accurate. The heart transplant program moves with carefully choreographed steps. The team—surgeons, cardiologists, pharmacists, nutritionists, social workers, coordinators – anybody involved with the transplant patient—meet every day at noon.

According to Dr. Dickinson, "We run the list of patients every day. We devise or alter strategies according to the patient's needs. It is important we leave the meeting with one clear plan for every patient. If, for instance, that plan calls for getting the patient out of bed and walking, then every team member who enters the room that day will reinforce that message. The nutritionist, the surgeon, the nurses—all will ask, "How many times did you walk today, Mike?"

Dr. Dickinson emphasizes that from the initial interview to discern if an individual is a viable candidate for a transplant, to the discharge of that patient after the surgery, candor prevails. "We don't sugarcoat the message. We bluntly discuss the risks."

I explained to Dr. Dickinson that I was never under consideration for "Patient of the Year." I was claustrophobic and suffered from an emotionally debilitating need to move, to get out of bed. I was consumed with stepping outside that confining room just to walk and regain some form of independence; to relieve the oppressive boredom of a hospital bed and four sterile walls. I was emotionally unhinged.

Dr. Dickinson points out there are different types of patients. After determining what a heart transplant entails, some simply say NO. They don't want to go through it. Others pay little attention to what we say; their response is "I want it. I want it." He goes on to say, "Patients who go through advanced procedures must have a desire to live; must have a reason to live."

Included in that daily meeting is a discussion of the patient's emotional health. Dr. Dickinson points out, "While the drive to live is critical, I'm apprehensive when it isn't there. I'm also concerned with the response to the question, 'What are you going to do after the transplant?' I worry about the passive patient, when there's just no fire. Patients who don't speak up trouble me."

Spectrum Health has become a leader in advanced heart and vascular care, ranging from prevention to heart and lung transplants. Countless lives are saved or extended every day.

I asked Dr. Dickinson, "Does it ever reach a point of routine, just another day at the office?"

The response to my question was quick and emphatic. "Never!" To emphasize his point, Dr. Dickinson told the story of his colleague, heart transplant surgeon Dr. Asghar Khaghani.

A heart transplant is complicated surgery requiring intense and unremitting concentration. The surgery can last anywhere from four to seven hours[26]. Dr. Khaghani had just completed one transplant and was relaxing in the cafeteria while preparing to do another; this would prove to be a 36-hour day for the distinguished surgeon. In between surgeries, Dr. Dickinson asked his colleague and friend, "Asghar, are you all right. Can I get you anything?"

Noting Dr. Dickinson's concern, Dr. Khaghani smiled and responded, "I am fine. This is why we are here."

Such was the residual adrenaline from the day's activities, that on the way home Dr. Khaghani was stopped for speeding.

To qualify as a transplant cardiologist, a requirement to go on three organ procurement runs must be met. It is a fore to aft professional and emotional experience. While one family gathers to say good-bye as the heart of their brain-dead loved one is harvested, another family and patient eagerly awaits the arrival of the heart and a new life. "You experience the total gamut of emotions," says Dr. Dickinson.

Dr. Dickinson recounts one of his runs. "I'm in the operating room and see the chest opened to reveal this beautiful beating heart that is about to be removed. The heart is gorgeous. We return to the side of the recipient in the operating room, healthy heart in tow, where meticulous preparations have been made and the surgery team awaits the healthy heart to begin the transplant. You need only compare the two hearts to know this is right. And you have to personally live it to know it is right."

Dr. Dickinson had some pointed words regarding my cardiologist and writing partner Dr. James. "There are two types of doctors," he says. "There are those who are brilliant with the books. And then there are the scrappers who have an abundance of common sense, and that common sense just might be more important. Mike James has that scrapper personality. He is a bigger than life persona in a hospital. He knows his patients, is passionate about his patients."

As this is written more than a year has elapsed since my transplant. It would be an understatement to say life is good.

---

26   I'm told my transplant took seven hours

Gone is the shortness of breath that severely impaired my mobility. Gone is the constant fatigue, the lethargy that hovered over the physical aspects of my life. Gone is begging off seeing good friends due to an inability to drive, and being too proud to ask them to pick you up. And gone is the constant dozing in that easy chair in the living room. For the record, I still grab an occasional nap in that chair, but now it is by choice.

I participate fully in the unique joy and caring that accompanies membership in a large family and having good friends. No longer am I treated with deference due to my condition. The transplant provides no special privilege when the trash-talking begins; the new heart is fodder for many tasteless and caustic remarks. I love it.

Excellence and class aren't the brick and mortar of an institution, rather it is the people who hold forth daily in that institution. I attribute the new stranglehold I have on life to the capable men and women who comprise the excellence that pervades the cardiovascular program at Spectrum Health.

After transferring my cardiac care to Spectrum Health I was frequently asked if I was comfortable leaving the vaunted cardio program at the University of Michigan. Not to demean the quality of care I received at the University of Michigan – it was superb in every way, as were the people—but the answer is a resounding YES, I am more than comfortable at Spectrum Health.

Just as the state of Michigan can boast two of the finest university educational and athletic programs in the country, two equally outstanding medical programs also share center stage.

The medical care I receive at Spectrum Health is nothing short of outstanding. Not only is it delivered with great expertise, but it is also encased in warmth and class. From the first visit with Becky the transplant coordinator that began the process, to my most recent visit to biopsy the new heart to determine if there is any rejection, I was always made to feel special.

My life has changed dramatically. Once again I know the sense of accomplishment that accompanies a well-crafted sentence. I know the joys of family, the laughter, the caring and the "I gotcher' back" assurance that means so much. I know the feeling of contentment in the week that follows a win by the Michigan State Spartans and the Detroit Lions.

The remaining years will be spent, writing, laughing, caring, and thanking God every day that I am able to do all three. That special relationship with the Lord will never be taken for granted again. Never.

I often wondered what thoughts occupy the minds of surgeons and their teams after performing a complicated, life-saving procedure. Do they step back for a moment and contemplate what just happened? Like Vince Lombardi's standard for success, are they able to survey the playing field and say, "I gave my best." Do they think about the patients and their families? Nothing will ever be the same for them again. Do they think about those who have preceded them – people like William Heberden, Andreas Gruentzig, Michael Debakey, and so many more. Or do they just want to get out of those wet scrubs and into a dry martini? I hope all of the above is true.

My final words are those of gratitude.

I once wrote, "I enjoy the support and love of two strong, independent, caring women. No man should be so blessed. Carol and Mara are my life's foundation." I see no reason to change a word of that sentiment.

I am also blessed with the love of a strong network of family and friends; brothers, sisters, aunts, uncles, cousins, nephews, and nieces. The calls and their collective irreverent sense of humor never fail to let me know how fortunate I am.

I am deeply indebted to the outstanding medical teams who extended my life. Their training and efforts, I assure you, will be honored by the knowledge they have added life to my years.

I am particularly grateful that Dr. Michael James has been a critical part of my cardiac care throughout the years. While the surgeons certainly stand out, there are others – the countless cardiologists, nurses (even though I needn't waste my time preparing an acceptance speech for "most beloved patient award"), the PA's, the dieticians, the occupational therapists, the physical therapists, the coordinators – to name a few is to surely overlook others, and that is not my intent. And a special salute to Gerhard, the nighttime custodian who always had a kind comment, an off-color joke, and who never failed to ask, "Can I get you anything, Mike?"

There is another poignant component to my story.

There was a time when my life consisted of watching television and sleeping, frequently done at the same time. I was not a father, a husband, a writer, and I had all but forsaken the once-cherished pastime of reading. I couldn't walk from one room to another without gasping for breath.

We each have certain responsibilities around our house. Two of mine were the weekly shopping and taking out the trash on Sunday nights, each according to his ability. Menial as the tasks were, I was unable to perform either one. Watching your wife take out the trash while you are sitting in an easy chair is an assault on personal dignity.

The cardiac communities of the University of Michigan and Spectrum Health worked miracles with my old and new heart. While I no longer gasp for breath and my activity level has increased significantly throughout the past few years, the real beneficiary has been my dignity. And I will never forget where I once was, and where I am today.

In the unlikely event that Dr. James precedes me in death, I will rise at his wake, glass in hand, and tell all that he fulfilled Dr. Stein's directive. His professional epitaph will read, "He added life to his patients' years. And did so with their dignity intact."

CHAPTER SIXTEEN

WHAT LIES AHEAD

"Twenty years from now you will be more disappointed by the things you didn't do than by the ones you did. So throw off the bowlines. Sail away from the safe harbor. Catch the trade winds in your sails. Explore. Dream. Discover."
—MARK TWAIN

Dr. Michael James:

Thoughts of a book of shared perspectives from cardiologist and patient regarding pivotal events in the ongoing care of a heart attack victim has long dominated my professional life.

I'd mentally craft a paragraph or two based on incidents that occurred during appointments in my cardiology practice. I'd fashion lists of topics for chapters while driving to and from work. I'd organize those chapters while traveling up north for a ski weekend. It was never far from the surface.

Now that I am in the twilight of my career, it's time to pause and put those thoughts to paper.

Mike Ranville was a natural to accompany me in exploring and implementing the project. He was in the right place at the right time. It seemed every time he needed something more than current technology could provide it became available—from medications, to tests, to tools.

His case underscores another theme coursing the pages of this book; quality heart care is not confined to status or wealth.

Neither Dick Cheney nor Mike Ranville is an anomaly. They are two heart patients who, while differing dramatically in celebrity, are alive today due to a marked similarity in access to recent advancements in the field of cardiac care.

Timing is everything, or, in our case, lousy timing was nearly debilitating. At the outset of my research I discovered that former Vice-President Dick Cheney wrote a book with his cardiologist, Dr. Jonathan Reiner. It was exactly the project I discussed with Mike. Even more upsetting, the Cheney-Reiner effort was very well done.

A HEART ATTACK IS NO LONGER A DEATH SENTENCE

We decided instead to focus on advancements in the field of cardiology through the years, citing famous heart patients as President Dwight D. Eisenhower and Vice President Dick Cheney. The heart attacks and subsequent recovery programs of Ike, Dick, and Mike underscore the availability of quality heart care to all, regardless of station in life. We tell our story by drawing on Mike's cardiac history and how my training and experiences dovetailed neatly with his needs.

Writing the book I became intrigued with the circumstances surrounding President Eisenhower's heart attack on September 23, 1955; it played a major role in shaping public opinion of heart disease. I concluded that not only was Ike misdiagnosed but the care he received was pedestrian at best. This was particularly evident in the critical first few hours, and extended into the first twelve hours. I've long believed that in today's litigious society if a patient received the diagnosis and initial care given to President Eisenhower, a lawsuit certainly would have been trotting close behind, a no-brainer for a hungry ambulance chaser. Yet Ike survived, served a second term, and played a lot of golf after his White House days. However simple and basic, there is still much to be said for diet and exercise.

Examining and comparing both the Cheney and Eisenhower cases with Mike's, allows for a clear illustration of how heart care has changed through the years and affords the opportunity to highlight the giant leaps in quality and availability.

I envision this book to serve as a patient guide. Hopefully if the turf-laden, special-interest-driven, woefully-complicated health care system is to survive and serve its patients, then more decisions and money must be put in the hands of those patients. Bluntly, too many tests are being conducted and too many drugs are being administered, draining the system of sorely needed financial solvency.

Not unlike education and assertions of, "The children are our only concern," a lot of people are leading comfortable lives under the guise of, "We're only doing what's best for the patient."

I continue to be amazed at the number of unnecessary tests conducted, and the vast array of tools patients are saddled with, that serve only to enhance the pocketbooks of those ordering them. Claiming the rationale underlying the ordering of those tests and installation of those devices is totally devoid of personal enrichment is medical sophistry at its worst.

I am extremely proud that our group, the Thoracic Cardiovascular Institute, demands an unequivocally honest brand of cardiology from its members. Such a notion was instituted early in my training and reinforced when I came to TCI. While serving in the leadership of our group and in the training of our Fellows, I have insisted that those rigidly high standards not be compromised. I make these statements not to enhance my own worth, or that of my partners, but to underscore there are those in the medical profession who are concerned about the abuses within the system. There is a problem and TCI isn't the only one aware of it.

The abuse of a few can easily taint the many competent, cost-conscious physicians who conduct their practices in an ethical and solid fashion. This is not unlike the political arena where the corrupt behavior of a small number can contaminate the hard work of honest elected officials who seek only to serve their constituents. Stories of physicians who line their pockets with proceeds garnered from excessive and unnecessary tests can infect public confidence in the overwhelming majority of principled physicians who practice honorable, disciplined, and caring medicine. Our already fragile health care system does not benefit from headlines such as, "THE $10M MEN OF MEDICARE," or "SEVEN PHYSICIANS, $93 MILLION."

Our current health care system is constructed to reimburse for things done to the patient. When a test is ordered, the ordering physician is reimbursed, not unlike inviting the fox to take up residence in the henhouse.

Cardiology will not be spared from scrutiny.

I can still recall a discussion on reimbursements I had with a classmate during my days as a student. We decided to make a list of the various specialties to determine who could order the most procedures that would directly benefit the ordering physician, who had the most "pop stands" as we called it. Unfortunately, we concluded it was the cardiologist.

Today, that discussion should be aggressively pursued.

How often does a patient need an EKG? Echocardiogram? Stress test? Nuclear stress test? Cardiac catheterization? Stent? Bypass surgery? ICD? Pacemaker?

It was not long ago that the quickest way to bilk the system was to set up an office, purchase a nuclear camera, and then order a nuclear test on almost everyone who came into your office.

Physicians rarely police other physicians, unless they are in the same group where pressure can be exerted to change questionable patterns.

Recently, TCI hired a physician formerly employed by a certain Dr. X who directed his subordinate to read tests in a slanted manner thereby creating a well-worn path to ordering the use of cardiac tools on unsuspecting patients, all ensuring the financial benefit of that ordering physician. The younger physician quickly recognized the inherent dishonesty of the process, but he still needed retraining when he joined our group.

Dr. X was investigated by Medicare and fined $2 million, the same amount levied against the hospital where the tests and procedures were conducted. Dr. X is still practicing.

Hospitals do not get a free pass. They are generously reimbursed for the procedures. As such they lack an incentive to address any effort to control those who indiscriminately order them, and, not surprisingly, are frequently lax in doing so.

Patients should be urged to join the battle. For instance, on the next visit to their cardiologist's office if, an EKG, stress test, echocardiogram, or 24-hour holter is ordered, ask who owns the equipment. More often than not the shallow response is, "Who cares? If it's covered by insurance that means it doesn't cost anything." That myopic and self-serving attitude, and it is a prevalent one, drives health care costs out of sight, and swells the pockets of those who claim to be doing "only what's best for the patient."

However, if the patient controls the purse strings, and that purse contains a finite amount of health care funds, the scenario is significantly altered. The patient now has a vested interest in questioning the ordering physician regarding the necessity and anticipated yield of, a certain test or procedure. It's very simple—and oh, by the way, doctor, who owns the equipment that will be used in that test or procedure?

Case studies are replete with the ordering of totally unnecessary tonsillectomies and hysterectomies for nothing more than highly suspect reasons.

One million prostates have been removed without so much as a nudge to the mortality rate needle. The true beneficiary of such hasty and questionable action is the Depends industry who reaps the financial rewards associated with treating the undesirable side effects. The prostate-specific antigen (PSA) as a screening test is on the way out.

We have good data to show that aggressive screening done back in the 1900's and early 2000s led to the diagnosis and treatment of over 1.1 million men, who, if they had never been tested, never been diagnosed, never been treated, were destined never to be bothered by their prostate cancer. The surgery results in impotence in as many as 40% of patients and incontinence in an equal number.

The medical community is capable of responding when pressure is exerted. For instance, the interval for colonoscopies, once every five years, is now once every ten years. Routine pelvic exams are now subject to greater critical scrutiny.

The cardiac arena sorely needs a thorough assessment designed to fashion realistic guidelines that govern the ordering of the vast arsenal of testing procedures at its disposal. Further, the expected yield of information needs to be balanced against the efficacy of the expensive and sometimes unnecessary tools that are routinely borne of those tests. Put another way, just because it's there doesn't mean it has to be used.

One of the "sacred cows" of cardiology, bypass surgery, comes to mind as an area begging for scrutiny. The usual standard of care is a yearly evaluation by the cardiologist. This, of course, includes a history and physical. A major reason for the visit is to determine if an inadequate supply of blood to a certain area is due to a blockage of blood vessels leading to that area – ischemia. Has there been a re-occurrence or new symptoms? The visit also allows for careful monitoring of risk factors; blood pressure, lipids, smoking, weight loss, and exercise. Medications also need to be evaluated.

If my patients have normal left ventricular function it needs occasional revisiting. I prefer to conduct an annual exercise test that allows me to gauge aerobic capacity, blood pressure response to exercise (comparing one year to another), and determine whether there is evidence of recurrent ischemia.

This fairly simple and relatively inexpensive test also gives the patient motivation to continue exercising and avoid being lectured at the annual visit; namely, have you been doing your aerobic exercise over the past year? If asked how much exercise is needed, I give 2 options and if the patient says, "I'm busy all day," that's a wholly insufficient response. Purchase a pedometer for about $10 and try to attain at least 10,000 steps per day. A better option is to sustain an aerobic activity. Options are simply walking at the same pace, treadmill, exercise bike, swimming, or if out of town on a business trip, walking the stairs will do, as long as the exercise is sustained. How often? At least three times per week, but preferably five with an appropriate warm up and cool down.

My patients are involved in their care, at least to the extent their ability to comprehend allows. I commonly tell them that the decision to move to the next level in their care—and contemplate use of one of the tools in our arsenal—is based on what they tell me and what I see.

It was common practice to do a yearly nuclear test, but BlueCross/Blue Shield recently changed their policy to allow the test only once every three years. Medicare still allows a nuclear test whenever the physician feels it is needed. Far too often, though, determining that need is driven by the proceeds on a profit and loss statement.

To illustrate, there was a physician practicing in the mid-Michigan area who employed a person who was given only one responsibility, monitor charts and determine when the next test could be ordered. To the surprise of no one, he owned all the equipment.

My patients are kept in the loop. In that regard, they are generally aware if a test is needed. At some point it's already been discussed. Since the test is normally covered by insurance, they readily approve.

That "whatever you say, doctor" frame of mind, though, can be fraught with problems. As a cardiologist I am privy to some of the abuses stemming from procedures involving stents and bypass surgery.

I can recall an incident that occurred when I was in a patient's room. The curtain was drawn but I could overhear the conversation in the next bed. The cardiac surgeon explained the patient's heart disease in this fashion:

"Well, sir, you have these narrowings in your heart that are like 'tiny bombs' that can go off at any time and cause a heart attack. But we can do surgery to fix the problem."

Total unmitigated garbage. But what is to be done when people in white coats with medical credentials, who gather at the foot of your hospital bed, during a period of stress in your life, proffer that kind of counsel?

So how is the vulnerable patient able to discern if the tinker toys, tools, or the lotions and potions being discussed are appropriate? Common sense should not be ruled out. Many patients are reluctant to ask what they deem to be difficult questions for fear of offending the doctor. If a difficult question offends the doctor, then it's time to find a doctor who is not offended by a difficult question, but welcomes it. If still not satisfied and the patient harbors even the smallest of suspicion regarding what is being proposed, then ask for a second opinion—especially if no improvement has been realized.

I welcome a request for a second opinion. While I know I took Mike by surprise when I was the one making the request, that second opinion increased his comfort level at a time when it was sorely needed. And despite tales of a "messiah complex," physicians are human and welcome another opinion—especially one that agrees with theirs.

Central to all health care is the physician-patient relationship.

When is the last time your primary care doctor or your cardiologist actually touched you, not inappropriately, but just a reassuring pat on the back that says, "I care about you, and your family?" Equally important, when is the last time your doctor made eye contact with you?

Much of the personal contact, so important to the physician-patient relationship has been sacrificed on the altar of computer efficiency. Whatever information is contained in that computer isn't going anywhere. It can be held in abeyance long enough for the physician to look up and acknowledge that a human being is in the room; someone in need of the physician's medical training, someone with a family who will hang on every word uttered by that physician, someone unsure of the future, someone who for weeks has had the date of the appointment circled on the refrigerator calendar. It's that important.

That patient's personal dignity warrants—demands—more than just a cursory nod when entering the room, followed by a recitation of the test results carefully noted in the computer, then concluding with a cavalier announcement that still another test is being ordered, "see staff on the way out for scheduling."

Sadly, throughout the computer-driven appointment – the appointment carefully circled on the refrigerator calendar, the appointment that represents the most important moment of the past few months in that patient's life – the physician barely concedes the existence of the patient. No pat on the shoulder to reinforce "You are important. We're doing all we can for you." No look of warmth accompanied by a smile to soothe the patient's anxiety. No personal question as to how the family is holding up under the changes brought on by the heart problem. Thankfully the National Center for Health Statistics is now tracking the time physicians spend with their patients during appointments. However, they warn, "With the new health care law ushering millions more into the system, time in the exam room might get even tighter."

These are all fixable problems. And it is why I am pausing to record observations, concerns, and noteworthy research that comprise my nearly fifty years as a cardiologist.

Some may be offended; so be it. I leave others to vie for the "Mister Congeniality" award.

Some may challenge my claims. I welcome the debate. On many of the issues I raise, the time to "drop the gloves" and have at it is long overdue.

Some may even welcome the points raised in the previous pages. Along with the offended and the debaters, we need to chart a productive course for the future to determine how to improve the state of cardiac care and do so with a critical eye on assignment of dwindling resources.

Again, I asked Mike Ranville, one of my patients throughout the years, to join me and offer his candid perspective of the advances realized in cardiac care. In the thirty years I have been his cardiologist he has never been reluctant to aggressively question my recommendations. To my delight he never "pulled his punches."

We need to know where we've been. There are some fascinating stories associated with the discovery and eventual deployment of the many tools at our disposal to treat heart patients. The trial and error, the stuttered beginnings, all plays a role in the ability to combat the nation's number one killer. It's time to discuss heart disease, and patients and their families – warts and all.

CHAPTER SEVENTEEN:

HEART DISEASE— THE GREAT EQUALIZER

"Except for the occasional heart attack, I never felt better."
—VICE-PRESIDENT DICK CHENEY

TOOLS OF THE HEART FAILURE SPECIALIST

Dr. Michael James:

Famous people have heart attacks. Some commendably parlay their celebrity to draw needed public attention to today's greatest killer.

Popular night time talk show host David letterman learned he had a clogged artery during a morning angiogram. Recalling that his father died of a heart attack at age 57, and keenly aware of the pivotal role played by genes in heart problems, Letterman underwent bypass surgery—that very afternoon. To his credit, he used his late-night bully pulpit to enlighten the national audience on heart disease.

After incurring a heart attack and then undergoing quintuple bypass surgery, long time talk show host and newsman Larry King became a strong advocate for the proper care and feeding of the heart, of good eating and exercise, as did former President Bill Clinton following his bypass surgery.

There are others who belong in the discussion but aren't readily associated with infirmities of the heart; people like Barbara Walters, Martin Sheen, Mike Ditka, Robin Williams and Jennie Garth. And while it has for the most part flown under the pen of historians, Winston Churchill is believed to have had a mild heart attack while visiting the White House in December, 1941, and another one in 1943 following a bout with pneumonia.

All of the above share one noteworthy thing in common. After learning of their heart problems, they continued to lead vibrant and productive lives.

Status and wealth provide no shelter from heart problems. Nor does status and wealth create a special path to privileged cardiac care. I take great pride in the fact that the citizens of Main Street, America, where the vast majority of my heart patients dwell, receive the same quality care as those who reside on Pennsylvania Avenue.

Interestingly enough, Mike Ranville's heart problems closely parallel those of Dick Cheney's. Both smoked, paid little homage to diet and professionally burned the candle at both ends. And both should have chosen their parents more carefully. Mike's journey back to health and productivity also paralleled Cheney's.

Both saw a significant and positive improvement in the quality of life after receiving a Left Ventricular Assist Device, known as an LVAD. Mike's heart, beating in the tiny mid-western community of Charlotte, Michigan, population 8,000, is powered by batteries, just as Dick Cheney's was when he navigated the politically sophisticated environs of power in Washington, D.C.

The lives of the rich and famous, and their heart problems, are well-documented. Whenever Dick Cheney and his well-known heart make an appearance on the evening news, his very able cardiologist Dr. Jonathan Reiner must sit back and smile with satisfaction at the attention heaped on his famous patient. And justifiably so. Dick Cheney's willingness to talk about his heart problems, coupled with the excellent care presided over by Dr. Reiner, has surely prompted others to seek medical attention.

While celebrities and their cardiologists have a more public encounter with heart disease, the vast majority of heart patients are common folk. Even though the progress of my patients isn't celebrated on the evening news, their successful treatment is a great source of satisfaction to me.

Whenever I undertake my now less-hectic commute home after work, I do so in the knowledge that my patients are leading gloriously normal lives; out walking the dog, playing ball in the park, laughing on the front porch with neighbors. While Dr. Reiner returned his famous patient to the post of "second most powerful man in the free world," I take great consolation in the fact that I have returned many of my patients intact to their families where they now enjoy those routine but unforgettable moments in life; football and soccer games, Christmas pageants, graduations, Bar Mitzvahs, First Communions and so much more.

Patients do care. At the 25th anniversary of his heart attack, Mike paused to send a note thanking me for the continuing education I regularly pursued that enabled him and my other patients to benefit from the most up-do-date cardiac care available. But he went further and placed his renewed life in context. He mentioned that many mundane aspects of his daily regimen that hold little interest to the outside world were now fundamental to him and his family. In his case, Mike mentioned the ability and willingness to read and write, "Two of God's greatest gifts never again to be taken for granted."

He thanked me for the opportunity that made it possible to compete in the marketplace, to provide for his family, to do things for them, to be a husband, a father.

He thanked me for the opportunity that rewarded him with a front row seat at his rather large family gatherings.

He thanked me for the opportunity that enabled him to make a contribution to society, an opportunity that gave him the ability to withstand the physical and mental rigors necessary to write a book. I learned he often arose at 4:30 a.m. to write, and then moved on to his normal hectic day. The book was well-received and went on to be a critical segment of a famous movie.

He thanked me for the opportunity that afforded an experience no one could ever take from him—being present when his daughter was awarded her Ph.D. He still speaks warmly of that moment when her advisor emerged from a meeting with the dissertation team and announced for all to hear, "Congratulations Dr. Ranville."

The cardiologist in me was grateful to have played a part in Mike's life. The grinder was moved.

Dr. Reiner may have had grip 'n grin pictures of himself and Dick Cheney on the walls of his office, but I have something just as precious; requests for my presence at wedding anniversaries that easily would not have occurred, invitations to family get-togethers celebrating a significant moment like a graduation or admission to the bar, books warmly inscribed with "Thanks for keeping me alive to write this." And so much more, all from patients and their families who truly appreciated my efforts.

The tools available to treat heart failure over the years have grown appreciably, both in quantity and quality. They've made it possible for cardiologists to become far more aggressive in both preventing further deterioration and restoring the defective parts. Those laboring outside the public eye in the cardiology research labs around the world deserve special mention. Each and every innovation is characterized by directly attacking the most difficult technical challenge possible and then employing the most sophisticated and creative engineering available to solve that problem.

Always keeping in mind, though, the parts fashioned by the Good Lord for the original version, are far superior to any replacements we devise.

The accounts reciting creation of the tools available to the heart specialist represent a fascinating story for the pages of history.

CARDIAC TRANSPLANT

Perhaps no other moment in the annals of cardiac care was more widely celebrated than the first heart transplant. The medical miracle was performed on December 3, 1967, by Dr. Christiaan Barnard.

A dynamic and photogenic forty-five year old South African surgeon, Barnard was more than equipped to handle the onslaught of publicity that assured history would properly record the moment. Headlines heralding the operation sprinted around the world, and Christiaan Barnard became an instant celebrity.

The heart was harvested from a young woman, Denise Darvall, the victim of an accident while crossing a street in Cape Town the previous day. The patient, Louis Washkansky, was a 54-year old grocer suffering from diabetes and incurable heart disease.

In an effort to suppress the immune system and prevent rejection of the transplanted heart, Washkansky was administered a combination of steroids, radiation, azathioprine, and actinmomycin C. However, those same drugs were also responsible for decreasing the body's ability to fight infection. And the world's first heart transplant recipient died of pneumonia 18 days after the transplant.

Barnard performed a second transplant a month later. The recipient, Philip Blaiberg, lived for 19 months.

The first transplant in the United States was performed on an infant by Dr. Adrian Kantrowicz on December 6, 1967, at Maimonides Hospital in Brooklyn, New York, only three days after Barnard's first landmark surgery. While the infant died shortly after, the surgery was successful and much was learned from the experience. The technique, in particular, was rapidly being perfected.

Dr. Norman Shumway performed the first adult heart transplant in the United States on January 6, 1968, at the Stanford University Hospital. As the success rate for the surgery, increased, longevity became the overriding issue. From 1968 to 1971 survival was close to 50% at six months and 30% at two years. Shumway was among the leaders in improving the surgical techniques involved in transplants.

Every innovation represented a major stride in improving the longevity rate. The most impressive and useful of the advancements found that instead of trying to take out the entire heart of the recipient and then connecting all six of the necessary contiguous vessels; the inferior and superior vena cava and the four pulmonary veins and the two atria were left in place and the back of the donor's heart was sutured to a cuff of the recipient's heart. The new procedure made the overall surgery easier but other challenges still presented themselves, chief among them preserving the donor's heart for transplant and perfecting the drugs used to combat rejection.

The results have been encouraging, but still laden with frustration. Currently, there are approximately 2,000 transplants in the United States each year. In Michigan three centers are authorized to perform transplants; The University of Michigan Hospital in Ann Arbor, Henry Ford Hospital in Dearborn and Spectrum in Grand Rapids. Yet there are at least 30 times more candidates than available donors.

The ten year survival rate for a transplant recipient is now close to 85%. Thus the industry has embarked on a quest to create a totally mechanical heart, the initial fruits of that effort being Ventricular Assist Devices (LVADs).

Currently, Michigan hospitals have implanted approximately 15,000 VAD devices. Patients have been living productively for 6-7 years.

In January, 2015, Dr. Jonathan Haft, of the University of Michigan Frankel Cardiovascular Center, took a giant step in alleviating the wait time for a transplant when he implanted an artificial heart in 24-year-old Stan Larkin and sent him home to spend Christmas with his family and to await a transplant. As battery technology improves, it will be accompanied by an ability to recharge the internal battery externally.

With time will surely come smaller and more sophisticated devices, a blessing for current VAD patients. But a better and more efficient VAD will still only address symptoms, i.e. relieving shortness of breath brought on by little or no exertion. Needed more than ever is a redoubling of effort urging people to stop smoking, to seize control of their own diet, to more effectively manage their diabetes, to actively pursue a daily regimen of exercise. In essence, our goal should be to reduce the demand for the VAD device. Sadly, though, a more sophisticated VAD device will be realized long before sorely needed life style changes.

VENTRICULAR ASSIST DEVICES (VADs)

Despite popular belief that the VAD replaces the pumping chambers of the heart, as the name implies it only assists the poorly functioning ventricle.

The engineers who developed the VAD were inspired by the Romans ability to pump water up a hill using the continuous flow found in the Arcadian pump. They invented a smaller version using the same principle.

Using the adapted version of the pump, a Teflon graft is positioned in the apex of the left ventricle and then placed directly into the ascending aorta. The pump then assumes the function of the left ventricle and provides oxygenated blood from the lungs to the rest of the body.

The process assumes the right ventricle is still capable of taking the un-oxygenated blood to the lungs where carbon dioxide is replaced by oxygen. Still to be dealt with were the technical challenges associated with powering the pump, which requires continuous power.

The power, it was decided, would be provided by two possible sources; an electrical outlet or battery power. Critical to the success of the VAD is the necessity of the patient being both independent and educated enough to care for this sophisticated and expensive device.

The most frequent complications derived from bleeding and infection stemming from the need for the patient to be anti-coagulated to prevent the pump from clotting and infection setting in due to the fact that the drive line is external.

The cost of the procedure dangerously approaches prohibitive, approximately $500,000 and requires a hospital stay of three weeks or longer. Further, the patient needs a family member, or the equivalent, who agrees to function as a support staff – guardian angel, really – and become familiar with the function of the device as well as the control panel.

Receiving the VAD represents a huge undertaking. And while the success of the procedure depends on the patient's ability and willingness to undergo many changes in life, the commitment of the family member— the guardian angel—is equally important.

The results have been nothing short of spectacular.

Where once the patient's quality of life was virtually non-existent, dominated by sitting in a chair barely able to breathe, or an inability to walk from one room to the next without encountering severe shortness of breath, dramatic changes were witnessed. Following the VAD procedure they were regularly pursuing the many activities that enriched their former lives—tennis, golf and a return to full employment.

Who qualifies? A simple rule-of-thumb is frequently employed to determine eligibility – does the patient have the energy to shower and dress in the morning without taking a break? If not, they are a candidate; an over simplification perhaps, but incredibly close to the truth.

Chief among the items to prevent and address heart disease is diet. If there is any one item under the control of the patient responsible for a healthier heart, it is diet. While we know daily exercise is beneficial it cannot be measured and quantified.

But frequently not even strict adherence to a heart-friendly diet can assure avoidance of heart issues.

I know of no greater anomaly that has dotted my 45 years of medicine than the far-too-often encounter between two patients. The first is a thin, diet-conscious, jogger sitting in the Intensive Care Unit being administered to after a heart attack. The second is an obese, diabetic couch potato, brought in because of chest pains, but is being discharged after a cardiac catheterization was completely normal. Probably just gas from a pizza.

There are no guarantees associated with the proper care and feeding of a healthy heart. The healthy life style, however, does decrease the incidents of heart disease exponentially. And we can quantify that genetics plays a key role in determining the health of a heart.

The tools available to the Heart Failure Specialist are effective. We know they have extended and improved lives. There are many options readily accessible to today's cardiologist that did not exist even one generation ago. But there is a downside and it's is gaining more traction every day.

First and foremost, deployment of the tools is expensive, in some cases so expensive that their use is prohibitive. This translates into an availability confined to only a small fraction of the population meeting stringent criteria of suitability for the devices. It has forced a narrowing of eligibility to a point where cardiac patients can be divided into two groups; those with normal ejection fractions and those with impaired ventricular function, both dealing with a measurement related to the percentage of blood that leaves the heart with each contraction. Tough decisions are forced. Based on availability of resources, a prognosis has surfaced suggesting the greater the ejection fraction—those with an ejection fraction of better than 30%—the greater the possibility of receiving a device.

History and experience also become key factors.

People are living longer. Those who received devices have seen their lives extended. Years ago, they would not be alive to crowd the eligibility rolls of younger patients seeking access to a finite supply of new devices. The older patients, however, have been kept alive by the technology of their time; stents, pacers, ICDs and Coronary Artery Bypass Grafts. And now, when the left ventricle begins to fail, understandably we look to the most recent innovations, like the VAD.

Moreover, the aging group has witnessed a reduced mortality rate in their segment of the population, traced in large part to improved pharmaceuticals. Bluntly, more sophisticated and effective medicine, coupled with growing expertise on the part of cardiologists, has translated into fewer deaths in the generation of Baby Boomers.

CHAPTER EIGHTEEN:

"Getting to the Root of the Problem—Keeping Arteries Healthy with Diet and Drugs"

"An Ounce of Prevention is Worth a Pound of Cure"

BENJAMIN FRANKLIN

David J. Strobl, DO, FLNA:

My friend and colleague, Dr. Michael James, asked me to pen a chapter on what I do best. I'm known in our practice as "The Lipid Guru."

For the record, Lipids are blood fats: cholesterol and triglycerides the most common ones. My job is to control them in order to prevent further injury to a patient's already damaged pump.

When Mike Ranville had his heart attack on September 23, 1984, I was a first year cardiology fellow at the Cleveland Clinic. At the time it was regarded as the premiere heart program in the world, a distinction it enjoys yet today.

Among the many significant contributions to the field of cardiology brought forth from the Cleveland Clinic, the heart catheterization procedure stands apart. Dr. James aptly described the results yielded in the catheterization lab as "critical to an accurate diagnosis and subsequent treatment program…the most important tool available to the interventional cardiologist."

The origin of the catheterization is as fascinating as its application.

Several years before I moved to Cleveland for my cardiology fellowship training, Dr. Mason Sones was one of many fashioning contributions that would become the Cleveland Clinic legend. He determined that dye could actually be injected into a coronary artery without killing the patient, a discovery central to the creation of the catheterization procedure. While Dr. James wrote of Dr. Sones' discovery in Chapter Five, as Paul Harvey would say—"here is . . . the rest of the story."

Dr. F. Mason Sones Jr. joined the Cleveland Clinic in 1950 at age 32. He was charged with establishing a cardiac imaging laboratory. In 1958, Dr. Sones was working in his basement cardiac laboratory on a 26-year-old patient with rheumatic heart disease. He was assisted by cardiologist-in-training Dr. Royston Lewis, a Welshman. They were attempting to perform an aortogram, a procedure where dye is injected into the main artery of the body to "light up" the artery with contrast to determine the presence of an aneurysm.

A gruff but talented cardiologist, Dr. Sones was not a poster-boy for cardiac care. He often performed procedures while a cigarette dangled from his lip. Sterile forceps held the lit cigarette which was placed on the edge of the instrument table so it would be always be nearby.

While loved by his patients, Dr. Sones could be irritable and demanding with his staff. Such was his demeanor and reputation that some nurses reportedly hid in the bathroom when he appeared on the floor for rounds. Not only was he critical of his colleagues, but also nearly anyone who crossed his path.

Dr. Lewis was on call the previous night and needed sleep, not the ideal credential for working with the often irascible Dr. Sones. Lewis's job was to push the "injector" button that would fill the large artery with contrast dye.

They experienced difficulty positioning the catheter and inadvertently placed the catheter tip into the man's right coronary artery. Dr. Sones mumbled and cursed; the sleep-deprived Dr. Lewis mistook the swearing for "inject!" To Dr. Sones's horror, a large amount of contrast dye was injected directly into the patient's right coronary artery. The contrast "lit up" the patient's coronary arteries, a phenomenon never before witnessed in a living patient.

Dr. Sones feared "this mistake" would initiate ventricular fibrillation, a life-threatening arrhythmia. Instead, the young patient's heartbeat stopped completely, a condition known as asystole. Dr. Sones reacted quickly and instructed the patient to cough; his rhythm immediately returned to normal.

At that very moment Dr. Sones realized a patient could actually survive such an injection. The ramifications for diagnosis and subsequent care for victims of heart disease, he quickly discerned, were astounding.

Armed with his discovery, Dr. Sones journeyed to Hollywood and convened a discussion with filmmakers on development of a camera and a process whereby moving picture films could be taken of the injection. With the filmmaker's expertise and assistance Dr. Sones developed the first catheterization filmmaking process, now known as a cineangiogram. He continued to refine the process, experimenting with smaller amounts of contrast dye that would increase the safety factor when injected into the arteries. The end result was the historic birth of the cardiac catheterization procedure.

Dr. Sones understandably became cardiac royalty. He received hundreds of awards and honors in his lifetime for what is considered one of the most important discoveries in the history of cardiology. However, he was a tireless and disciplined perfectionist; his family life and his health suffered. Consumed by his work, he became even more ill-natured and surly and divorced in 1963. His tobacco habit worsened; in1981 he suffered a brush with lung cancer. Still he would not, could not, stop smoking.

When I arrived for training at the Cleveland Clinic in 1983, Dr. Sones was recently retired, although he still kept an office in the Cardiology Department where he would read and write. Rarely seen, he avoided conversations with my fellow trainees and never attended or gave any lectures or grand rounds. He had a recurrence of his lung cancer in 1984 that resulted in the removal of a lung. His health deteriorated.

I had one, single, memorable glimpse of Dr. Sones early one morning at the Clinic. It was in the spring of 1985, he was unlocking his office door. Although only 66, he was gaunt, appeared much older, and was bald from chemotherapy. His days were numbered.

I finished my Cardiology training at the Cleveland Clinic on June 30, 1985. Sadly, I learned Dr. Sones died at home just two months later on August 29. My brief encounter of Dr. Sones that early morning is an image that will always be with me.

In one of life's great but totally misplaced ironies, the "Father of Modern Cardiology," the man who gave millions of patients extended lives with their families with his breakthrough procedure, was felled by a habit that is one of the biggest risk factors of the disease he worked endlessly to cure.

DIAGNOSIS AND TREATMENT

When I was studying at the Cleveland Clinic in 1984, they enjoyed the vaunted, world-wide reputation of unmatched excellence when diagnosing and treating heart disease. Heads of state, royalty, political notables, icons of the entertainment industry—all came to Cleveland for diagnosis and treatment of failing hearts. And to the Clinic's credit, to that list add Joe Six Pack and his family. Admission was based not on power or fame, rather a need for cardiac care.

Most of the referrals to the Cleveland Clinic were from outside institutions; very little inpatient or outpatient risk factor counseling was performed.

Enter Dr. Gordon Blackburn, a PhD from the East Coast. Dr. Blackburn was recruited to create the cardiac rehab program at Cleveland

Clinic. We became friends, a keen interest in cardiac rehabilitation on my part one of the positive byproducts of the friendship.

When I was training there in 1985 I found it amazing that the high normal cholesterol at the Cleveland Clinic hospital was 300 mg/dL. The "statin" drugs still awaited approval and not available at that time. Only a gritty mix called cholystyramine, and high doses of niacin, a water-soluble B vitamin, that caused uncomfortable flushing among other side effects, were on hospital formularies. Treating cholesterol was considered a nuisance and rarely addressed.

I joined the Thoracic and Cardiovascular Institute in 1987. One of our founding members, Dr. Wally Baird, was director of the cardiac rehabilitation program at the time Mike Ranville was recovering from his heart attack. I was asked to be the co-director of the program and, upon Dr. Baird's retirement, was tapped to lead it.

In 1988, an Expert Panel met in Bethesda Maryland and wrote the first "Adult Treatment Panel (ATP) Guidelines" for managing high cholesterol. Prior to this, it was not unusual for high normal cholesterol levels to reach up to 340 mg/dL or higher. Studies, such as the one conducted by Ansell Keys "Seven Countries Study," established a convincing link between high cholesterol and coronary events. The new cholesterol guidelines suggested that low density lipoprotein, LDL, or "bad guy cholesterol" should be lowered to less than 130 mg/dL.

Within the cardiac community, especially in the early stages, the guidelines were not without controversy. One of our biggest obstacles was 'This is not the way we've always done it."

The American Heart Association, to their credit, recruited and dispatched experts to take the podiums at hospital and medical conferences and explain the new guidelines and treatment protocols. I was asked to assist in the "Physician Cholesterol Education Program," and travelled throughout the country to introduce the new guidelines to practicing physicians. The talks were well-received and I take great pride in the fact that I was cited by the AHA for educating the largest number of physicians in the Midwest. The accolades paled, though, when placed alongside the discernible and improved quality of care afforded heart patients.

Treatment options were limited when the initial guidelines were first released. However, the statins, the much more potent LDL lowering drugs, were now available. The statin drugs caused dramatic lowering of LDL cholesterol. Many clinical trials confirmed that they not only lowered a patient's numbers, but also significantly lowered risk of a first or subsequent heart attack.

Developed and approved by the FDA, the first statin drug was released in 1989. Mevacor (Lovastatin) was followed by Zocor (Simvastatin), and then the blockbuster drug Lipitor (Atorvastatin). An even more potent statin, Crestor (Sosuvastatin), was introduced in 2003, and is now available in generic form.

Five years after the initial cholesterol guidelines, a second report was released that recommended even more aggressive LDL lowering in patients that have documented coronary artery disease. The guidelines have continued to evolve, and now most experts feel LDL cholesterol should be aggressively lowered to less than 70 mg/dL in high-risk patients such as Mike.

In 2015, new injectable cholesterol lowering drugs called PCSK9 inhibitors were approved for use in select high risk patients who do not achieve their cholesterol lowering goal despite being on a maximally tolerated dose of statin. These very expensive agents are actually human monoclonal antibody therapies that preserve an individual's LDL receptors, which clear the bad guy LDL cholesterol from the blood. One preserved receptor can thus recycle up to 150 times, clearing the blood of LDL cholesterol. These agents can incredibly reduce LDL by an additional 65% above and beyond what is achieved with background statin therapy.

In a large clinical trial completed in 2016, a significant reduction of cardiac events, including heart attacks and hospitalizations, was achieved compared to placebo therapy thus establishing these amazing biologic agents as an important new option in reducing cardiac events in high risk patients. In this trial, LDL cholesterol was lowered on average to 30 mg/

dl, suggesting that even more aggressive cholesterol lowering should be considered in patients with advanced coronary artery disease.

Although statins and PCSK9 inhibitors are clearly life-saving drugs, it is important to remember that diet is still the cornerstone of therapy for any cholesterol or triglyceride abnormality. Many of the patients I see in consultation for the first time are frequently on the correct medical therapy, but have never been counseled on a proper diet. The patients that have abnormal blood fats frequently have a genetic problem where their bodies cannot clear the abnormal particles.

I explain to these patients that they are born with only so many dump trucks to clear out the garbage. Medicines, such as statins, may help increase the number of dump trucks to some degree. However, if they still take in too much garbage the beds of the trucks will overflow and the result is elevated blood fats that can't be cleared.

If too much LDL cholesterol is present, it will sneak into the wall of the artery through exposed gaps. Once inside the artery wall, the LDL cholesterol initiates an inflammatory reaction which ultimately leads to the development of a plaque which is commonly known as atherosclerosis or hardening of the arteries.

Of greater concern is the process by which the thin covering over the plaque becomes inflamed and ruptures which leads to an instant clotting reaction and occludes the artery resulting in a heart attack. When the muscle of the heart is not receiving blood flow and oxygen, its cells literally die, which is commonly known as a myocardial infarction or heart attack. The more muscle the artery supplies, the more damage there is to the heart. The decreased pumping function of the heart is what leads to heart failure, and coronary artery disease is the number one reason why patients will develop heart failure.

YOU ARE (AND WILL BECOME) WHAT YOU EAT

So what is the most heart healthy diet to prevent the progression of coronary artery disease?

That answer in part depends on whether the goal is to lower cholesterol or triglycerides – or both. In many patients, the main goal is to lower their LDL cholesterol level. In that case, the most important dietary measure is to lower a certain type of fat called saturated fat.

There are three major dietary sources of fat: saturated fat, polyunsaturated fat, and monounsaturated fat. Saturated fat contains the main building blocks for the production of LDL cholesterol in the body. It is found commonly in red meat, dairy products, and baked goods.

The best way to determine the saturated fat in a packaged food is to read the food label attached to the product. I ask patients to become a student of the food label, and in particular to pay close attention to the amount of saturated fat listed. Another culprit is a manufactured fat called trans-fat. Trans-fats are "super saturated", fats that manufacturers add to products to maintain their stability and flavor. They are found in products such as stick margarine, baked goods, and fried foods.

Ideally, I like patients to eliminate as much saturated fat and trans-fat in their diet as possible. Therefore, I tell them to choose food items that contain the least amount of saturated fat as possible. It is not always possible to find an item with saturated fat content of "zero", but in that case I would try to get an item with a saturated fat content as close to "zero" as possible. A level of 0.5 grams to 1.5 grams per serving is acceptable. I don't ask patients to carry around a calculator to determine how much daily saturated fat they are consuming. Instead, I want them to follow the general rule of limiting saturated fat as much as possible.

It is not necessary to eliminate or limit all fat from the diet. We need a certain amount of dietary fat to maintain a normal blood fat metabolism. Therefore patients should not necessarily focus on low fat. Monounsaturated fats are heart healthy fats that will not raise your LDL cholesterol and will maintain a good level of HDL (high density lipoprotein) which is your protective or Good Guy cholesterol in the body. Your HDL helps transport damaging LDL cholesterol from the artery wall to the liver to dispose of it. Patients with higher HDL levels have a lower incidence of coronary artery disease. HDL can be improved through aerobic exercise and weight loss.

Monounsaturated fats can be found in olive and canola oil, almonds, avocados, and chickpeas (hummus). They are staples in the so-called Mediterranean Diet, proven in studies to lower heart disease risk. It is also reasonable to include some polyunsaturated fats in the diet such as corn oil and safflower oil. Fatty fish—salmon, herring, sardines, and tuna— also provide other essential fatty acids such as omega-3, proven to reduce the risk of fatal heart attacks and sudden cardiac death caused by electrical problems in the heart. Eating fish also has the positive effect of reducing the risk of stroke as well. Fish also contain other nutrients such as vitamin D, selenium, and other healthy proteins.

Triglycerides are another packaged blood fat that serve as a fuel source for muscles. You may remember the famous comedian/actor Rodney Dangerfield who starred in the film Caddyshack. In his stand-up routines, Dangerfield would always lament that he "got no respect." Well, I consider triglycerides as the Rodney Dangerfield of blood fats: many times they "get no respect" and are often ignored by treating physicians and patients. It is cholesterol and LDL cholesterol that get most of the attention-grabbing headlines. However, when triglycerides are over-produced and/ or not cleared properly in our blood streams, they also pose a cardiac risk that may in some patients be as important (or more important) as elevated LDL cholesterol.

Not all patients have elevated triglycerides. Some have a marked genetic disturbance where the triglycerides are so elevated (over 800 mg/ dl) that they put the patient at risk for pancreatitis, a condition where small vessels are blocked by the large fat globules in their bloodstream thereby preventing the pancreas from getting enough blood and oxygen. The pancreas becomes dangerously inflamed and the patient frequently goes into shock with their life in danger.

Many other patients have only mild or moderate elevations of their triglycerides. Triglyceride levels over 150 mg/dl but under 500 mg/ dl do not put the patient at risk for pancreatitis, however could pose a significant cardiac risk to the patient. Many times, more mild elevations of triglycerides may be ignored by physicians, since they are more concerned about managing LDL cholesterol. However, there are several reasons why triglycerides pose a threat to your arteries.

First, there is an inverse relationship between triglycerides and HDL (Good Guy) Cholesterol. As triglycerides climb upwards, HDL cholesterol will begin sneaking downwards. Conversely, the lower the triglycerides are maintained with diet, exercise, and weight loss the higher the HDL cholesterol affording protection to the arteries. Remember, HDL helps transport damaging LDL from the artery wall to the liver where it is removed from circulation.

Second, higher triglycerides will actually change the shape and size of LDL cholesterol, making these particles smaller and denser. The small "BB-like" particles are able to penetrate the artery wall much easier, causing inflammation and plaque. On the other hand, as triglycerides drop below normal, the LDL particles become larger and more beach ball-like, and are much less dangerous. Some physicians order particle size testing to determine a patient's added risk; however I believe that the triglyceride level is a good surrogate marker for the size of the LDL particle—and is included in a standard lipid blood test.

Therefore, like LDL cholesterol, I believe that lower is better when it comes to triglycerides. In some patients with dangerously high triglycerides, medical therapy with a class of drugs called fibrates is necessary. Prescription fish oil, which is both purified and concentrated compared to over the counter preparations, can also be helpful. However, for most patients, triglycerides can be lowered through diet, weight loss (particular around the waistline), and aerobic exercise.

So what in the diet can contribute to higher triglycerides? Similar to LDL cholesterol, a diet high in saturated fat and trans-fats can raise triglycerides. Although they have no effect on LDL cholesterol, simple carbohydrates can trigger significant triglyceride elevations in susceptible individuals. Not all carbohydrates are created equal. Complex carbohydrates are generally high in dietary fiber; they are the more heart-healthy carbohydrates and can be found in whole grains, brown rice, and vegetables (except potatoes). The term "simple carbohydrates" refers to refined carbs that the body immediately converts into sugar in the blood stream.

I instruct patient who are trying to lower their triglycerides to "avoid anything white." That includes white bread (or white flour foods), white rice, white potatoes, white pasta, and particularly white sugar. I also warn patients to be exercise caution regarding hidden sugars found in breakfast cereals, natural sugars (such as fruit juice, dried fruit, honey, molasses, and brown sugar), sugared beverages (such as soda, lemonade, sweetened iced tea), candy, cookies, and other baked goods.

Instead, I ask patients to substitute more complex carbohydrates for the simple carbohydrates in their diet whenever possible. For example: whole grain bread for white bread; yams/sweet potatoes instead of white potatoes; whole wheat or high fiber pasta instead of white pasta; brown rice instead of white rice; and zero calorie sweeteners instead of sugar.

The food label again is the best guide to lowering the simple carbohydrates in the diet. Just as we tried to limit the saturated and trans-fats on the label, I suggest trying to keep "sugar," listed under "Carbohydrates" on the label, as close to zero as possible. It does not translate into elimination of all carbohydrates, just the triglyceride raising simple carbohydrates. Foods high in dietary fiber are desirable and do not need to be avoided.

Most patients do not like the term "diet." I don't blame them – seems restrictive. However, the diet I describe is more of a substitution diet. The goal is to substitute foods that are lower in saturated fat and simple carbohydrates in the overall meal plan. The substitution plan does not mean perpetual hunger; it enables eating well. And can lower blood fats to desirable levels.

A SAMPLE SUBSTITUTION PLAN

So what would an ideal meal plan for a patient with coronary artery disease?

BREAKFAST: Mom was right. Breakfast is the most important meal of the day and should not be skipped.

Oatmeal is a good source of complex carbohydrates, and contains soluble fiber. Soluble fiber is soft and sticky, and absorbs water to form a gel-like substance inside the digestive system. It also binds to substances like cholesterol and sugar, preventing or slowing their absorption into the blood stream. It thus can help regulate blood sugar levels, and protect against heart disease by lowering blood cholesterol. I would avoid adding cream and table sugar for topping the oatmeal but instead substitute skim milk, fresh berries and/or a sugar substitute such as Splenda, Equal or Stevia.

If you prefer a cold cereal, avoid sugar-laden brands such as kids' cereals. Again, the food label is your guide. Try to find a whole grain cereal with limited sugar. At face value, Raisin Bran seems a good choice. However, it has 18 grams of sugar per cup. Most of us will have a larger bowl than one cup; therefore even more sugar. Dried fruit is like eating candy for someone with high triglycerides. Patients sometimes report that they are eating shredded wheat for breakfast. But under cross-examination they admit it is really Frosted Mini Wheats. Although a good source of fiber, I would counsel against the sugared variety. Instead, eat simple shredded wheat with skim milk, berries, and/or an artificial sweetener. Walking down the cereal aisle at the grocery store and comparing labels is helpful in finding a cereal that meets the goal of higher fiber/lower sugar.

One of my personal favorites is a whole grain waffle (frozen then toasted) topped with almond butter. Almond butter is lower in saturated fat than peanut butter, and is very high in the healthier monounsaturated fat. Thomas Multigrain Light English muffins are another excellent choice for complex carbohydrates and give eight grams of fiber per muffin.

Substituting egg whites for whole eggs is an excellent source of protein with no saturated fat. Egg Beaters are simply colored and flavored egg whites. Scrambled egg whites would be fine every day of the week. If the inner-chef beckons, an omelet could be fashioned. However, substitute fat-free or reduced fat cheese. No limit on vegetables, but higher fat and sodium-laced breakfast meats are to be avoided.

Some patients enjoy a glass of juice for breakfast; however, many juices are very high in concentrated sugar and are no different than drinking sugared pop that has high triglycerides or blood sugars. For example, an 8 ounce glass of orange juice has 24 grams of sugar. A similar serving of prune juice has 42 grams of sugar. I would instead substitute a light version of juice. Tropicana Light Orange Juice has 10 grams of sugar and Minute Maid Light Lemonade has only 4 grams of sugar. Although lower in sugar, V8 Vegetable Juice is very high in sodium, and should be avoided for most heart failure patients.

LUNCH: The sandwich will always be among America's favorite choices for lunch. And there is no reason why it can't remain so. Simply substitute a whole wheat or multigrain bread for white bread, and choose a lower saturated fat luncheon meat. Turkey and chicken are generally lower in fat, but even some deli ham can limit saturated fat to one gram per slice. The food label again is the best guide, and will also help identify lower sodium options and aid in avoiding higher fat choices such as bologna and salami.

Soups are frequently higher in sodium and should be avoided by heart failure patients. However, home-made soups, particularly those where the sodium can be controlled, can be a tasty and healthy option. Creamed soups should be avoided, unless they are made with skim milk. Vegetable, chicken, and turkey are good choices.

Homemade vegetarian chili is a good source of protein and fiber. I would substitute ground turkey (particularly 100% white meat available in the Jenny O's brand) for ground beef—or at least minimize the red meat. Limit or avoid cheese – unless fat-free or reduced fat.

Even "fast food" can be a healthy choice if you pick the right item on the menu. All establishments should have nutritional information in their store or on-line. Subway has many excellent choices. Substitute whole grain bread and choose meat and toppings that are low in saturated fat. Avoid cheese and mayonnaise but load up on veggies. Even (gasp) McDonald's and Wendy's now offer salads and grilled chicken options. Again, ask to hold the cheese and higher fat dressings.

Try to substitute a zero calorie beverage and avoid sugared pop and sweetened ice tea. Many places offer unsweetened herbal tea, which is quite good when iced.

DINNER: Don't bail out now. Dinner can be just as healthy and tasty as breakfast and lunch. A wide variety of foods are available for dinner, as long as the general rules of low saturated fat and reduced sugar are not abandoned.

Red meat, sadly a staple of the American diet, has much higher saturated fat than other sources of animal protein. I encourage patients to limit red meat; but again, there are options.

Small portions of lean red meat can occasionally be included on the menu plan. Caution must be exercised, though. Certain types of red meat, such as bacon, sausage, ribs, and lamb are particularly high in saturated fat and should be avoided all together. Pork chops, falsely advertised as "the other white meat," are high in saturated fat as well. Lean pork tenderloins may be the exception. And venison can be quite lean. Another option is bison or ostrich; both are similar in texture and taste to red meat but are actually lower in saturated fat than turkey.

The preferred, much healthier, and lower saturated fat option is poultry—namely chicken and turkey—as well as almost all fish, including shellfish such as shrimp and scallops. As mentioned earlier, even "fatty" fish such as salmon, herring, sardines, and tuna are actually very low in saturated fat but also provide other essential fatty acids such as healthy omega-3 fats.

Not to be overlooked is the importance of meal preparation. Avoid frying. Instead bake or grill with a little olive oil. If sautéing is required, choose canola or olive oil for cooking.

A stir fry is an excellent way to limit meat and include a variety of fresh vegetable. Substitute brown rice for white rice whenever possible. If ordering Chinese food, avoid breaded and fried items in your dish. Experiment with tofu, which is a good source of vegetable protein that is low in saturated fat.

Pasta dishes can be heart healthy, but be careful with cheese and consider marinara sauces over heavy cream items. Substitute whole wheat or high-fiber pasta when possible.

Fill up on steamed or raw vegetables, but be careful with butter and sauces. Consider substituting a squeeze of lemon juice on steamed vegetables instead of butter. Avoid white potatoes, but yams or sweet potatoes are high in fiber and quite filling. Watch out again for butter or brown sugar which negates many of the benefits of the healthier choices.

Pizza violates most of the rules since it is generally made with white flour and is high in saturated fat when the cheese and meat toppings are added. Dietary Science has yet to fashion a substitute for the "meat lovers" pizza. Don't let your taste buds even contemplate it—it's definitely off the list. However, some pizza dough now being tossed is made with whole wheat crust. Ask for only a sprinkling of cheese or consider trying a "cheese-less" pizza so you can still enjoy the pizza sauce flavor with the toppings. Substitute chicken or even lean ham for the pepperoni and sausage, and don't discount a handful of vegetable toppings instead.

Dining out with family or friends can be, and should be, a delightful experience. It is still on the table, just eat healthy. Consider incorporating some of the menu items and substitutions discussed above that are lower in saturated fat. We live in a society that is becoming more aware of the importance of proper diet. Don't be reluctant to ask for the courtesy of a special preparation from the kitchen. Most establishments are willing to accommodate dietary needs.

DESSERTS: Desserts can unfortunately undo many of the healthy choices incorporated into the entire diet. Most are laden with saturated fat and sugar. If high triglycerides are not a problem, and there is no need to limit sugar, low fat sherbet or frozen yogurt is a great desert. Again, fresh fruit topped with Splenda or Stevia is also a great way to top off a meal.

There are many more choices now in the grocery store for low fat and low sugar items such as frozen desserts and cookies. Become a student of the food label, and you will find some items you can still enjoy.

In summary, a healthy diet, one that does not endanger the arteries, is not a one-way trip to bland. Most people are on some semblance of a schedule that includes the same meal rotation each week. The key is to find menu items that can be substituted into the rotation that are both enjoyable and represent a healthy choice. There are numerous sources for recipes that are tasty but low in saturated fat and sugar. Don't be fooled by the shallow promises of fad diets. The approach I've outlined above is the product of solid research and success. It works. And, if adhered to, can dramatically lower cholesterol and triglyceride levels.

Remember, there are no rewards or punishments when it comes to lifestyle—just consequences!

Bon Appétit!

CHAPTER NINETEEN:

WHAT DOES
IT ALL MEAN?

"Hide not your talents, for use they were made.
What's a sundial in the shade?"
—BENJAMIN FRANKLIN

Parting Remarks: Dr. Michael James:

As I reflect on the cardiac history of Ike, Dick, and Mike, what comes to mind is not their time in the winner's circle; rather, it is the health enabling them to vigorously pursue the accomplishments that warranted their appearance in that winner's circle.

Many of my friends are retired from successful jobs; banking, engineering, as well as educators and, businessmen. They frequently ask why I don't retire, a question I have on occasion asked myself.

The truth is I absolutely love what I'm doing. Playing a key role in restoring patients' health and then watching as they once again become contributors to society, to their workplace, to their family—it just doesn't get old.

Not every patient is as fascinating as Mike Ranville. But every fifteen minutes I make a decision that affects a life that in turn affects countless

251

other lives. Most of these decisions are fairly direct for me, but as Malcom Gladwell explained in his classic book *Outliers*, it takes repetition of a task ten thousand times to do it well. It can be something as mundane as kicking a soccer ball, hitting a baseball, writing a proper sentence, or involve far more complicated and consequential actions such as making a diagnosis of palpitations, recommending an ICD, a Cardiac Catheterization, an LVAD, a heart transplant.

There is no substitute for the warm and collective embrace of a family thanking you for helping their loved one.

I've always felt the greatest accolade bestowed on a physician occurs when other physicians or those close to you personally, seek you to be their doctor. In that regard, neighbors, friends, and colleagues have regularly sat in my office seeking medical counsel. Being able to help them with both major and minor medical issues is one of my life's greatest joys.

A while ago a long-time friend came in for a pre-op evaluation prior to hip replacement surgery. While I had been managing his blood pressure, a pre-op EKG was necessary. One of our Medical Assistants did the EKG. When reviewing it I detected a prior heart attack. I reviewed the chart and sure enough, the EKG taken one year ago was different—no evidence of a heart attack.

Given that 10 percent of all heart attacks are silent, I started questioning my friend regarding any symptoms that could have been misconstrued by him. No such thing, he said. I started to tell him that we might need a stress test before approving him for his hip replacement and although he was outwardly calm, his face reddened. My comment had struck a sensitive nerve.

I took quick stock of the situation. Years of reading EKGs told me there are certain common mistakes that a novice EKG technician can make; it's simple, for instance, to switch the right and left arm leads but that was not the pattern noted on this EKG. I then walked out into the hall and said, "Ladies, make me happy and redo the EKG." Another MA happened to be sitting there and redid the EKG – completely normal. The first MA had not put the leads on correctly and if I had not looked at ten thousand EKG's prior to this one it might have set off a firestorm.

Insignificant decision? Probably. But every decision is significant to someone. Later, while driving home and mentally sifting through the events of the day, my thoughts drifted to Malcolm Gladwell as I figuratively read EKG ten thousand and one and was able to inform the patient (in this case a good friend) that there was no need for concern. The EKG had not been administered correctly, an immaterial event when considered in the context of a universe brimming with war and homelessness, but not to that patient and his family.

It's the adrenaline from the everyday decisions, the so-called uneventful ones, as well as the more consequential—that keep me from turning my life over to a rod and reel. No matter how well they are biting that day, my mind would still be back in a cramped room, reading the results of an EKG to an anxious patient and family.

Upon reflection, I am truly an Outlier, blessed with the opportunity and ability to make life-and-death decisions for patients and friends, and, most importantly, armed with the training and experience to translate those decisions into an improved quality of life. While some would say "right place at the right time," mine was not a smooth voyage. I bear the scars, and the physical and emotional calluses, incurred in that journey to the "right place at the right time."

I was turned down for the best high school in Cleveland—St. Ignatius—but my dad intervened and petitioned the Jesuits to give me a chance—just a chance. Dad was not easily dismissed, and they relented. I rewarded their gamble and dad's faith in me. I did well.

After St. Ignatius, despite a valiant effort, I was not accepted into either of the colleges of my choice, Georgetown or Notre Dame. Instead I settled for another Jesuit school, the University of Detroit. I did well.

I did not get into the medical school of choice. Refusing to be dissuaded, I opted for osteopathic school. Dr. Ward Perrin and Dr. Park Willis, both of whom played major roles in my medical training, felt if given the chance I could become a decent cardiologist. I did well.

I wanted to become a key influence to many students, interns, and residents, and to be a pivotal factor in the training of thirty-eight cardiologists. I did well.

I learned a great deal on my journey. The experiences are pivotal to what drives me today. When I hear some of my colleagues whining and moaning about how hard they work or how bad their day was, my threshold of sympathy is barely tolerable. When their complaining reaches the egregious stage I find it difficult to disguise my disgust and have, on occasion, "called them out." They don't know what a hard day is.

Not long ago I was attending a medical meeting. The day was done and I was relaxing with a cocktail. The person next to me asked, "Are you Dr. James?"

"Yes I am."

"You probably don't remember this but I sure do. I was a student of yours and on this particular day we happened to be heading into the cath lab at the same time. You told me that whenever you go into a procedure, you should have a little sweat in your armpits."

I do recall imparting that earthly counsel to my students. It was a way of stressing the importance of being focused; a little nervousness was good because it underscored the need for increased concentration. "First and foremost," I told them, "the cardinal rule is, do no harm. However routine to you, the procedure at hand is not routine to your patient."

I laughed. The sweaty armpits reference was a colorful way of invoking an image to make my point. If someone remembered it years later, it had certainly served its purpose.

I learned my former student was now a gastroenterologist. He volunteered, "Every time I do a scope, I have a little sweat under my arms. Just wanted to say thank you."

This was totally unexpected, but totally appreciated. This old grinder just smiled and humbly, but proudly, nursed his cocktail. Some moments in life are worth savoring. I was leaving my fingerprints on the next generation of healers; what a great sense of accomplishment.

Working with Mike on this book has also become an unexpected pleasure.

Being able to revisit highlights of my years as a cardiologist, some of which are mentioned above, is certainly personally rewarding. But they are included here not because I seek applause from my peers or patients; but, rather, to emphasize that the residue of seeking excellence, and doing so by putting the patient first, is a grand reward unto itself. If a grinder like Mike James can do it, so can anyone. Hopefully, that message will resonate with those who will be replacing me.

Mike keeps telling me that in order to craft an effective message I need to leave part of myself on the playing field we have created to tell our story. While I agonized over the fine line between boasting and inspiring, I concluded there are those in medical school, struggling with their studies, who just might find some solace and inspiration in the recounting of my journey as a grinder.

In that regard, not long ago I received a text message from a former student. A few years earlier I had written a letter of recommendation for him to get into Osteopathic Medical School. When the time came I successfully petitioned the internal medicine program director to accept him for an internal residency. Then I took him as a Fellow in my cardiology program. I was always fond of him. He wasn't gifted but worked as hard as any student I ever had—definitely a grinder.

Our exchange of texts:

He wrote: "Passed my cardiology boards. Thanks for all your support over the years."

I responded: "Good job. Yea. It's been a good run watching kids like you mature into competent cardiologists. Hope your training allows you to be successful.

He wrote back: "My training has prepared me well. You should be proud to have such an impact on so many cardiologists coming from your mentorship."

I was moved. Unbeknownst to him, pausing briefly to share a major moment in his life became a major moment in mine.

The patient perspective provided by Mike just might prompt other patients to overcome the inherent intimidation of dealing with a "messiah in a white coat" and ask some poignant questions about their treatment.

I've learned Mike is a bit of a grinder himself.

I ran into one of Mike's former colleagues, Scott, at a birthday party for a neighbor. I mentioned that Mike and I were writing a book together. He immediately recalled the name of Mike's first book.

When we were contemplating this effort I remember asking Mike when he found the time to write that first book. He was working a job that put unusual demands on his time. He said he used to rise at 4:30 a.m., write for a few hours, go to work, come home, and then write for an hour or two before going to bed. And he did so on a regular basis. Save for a time-out to watch a football game or two weekends were spent at the keyboard.

All this from a guy who'd had a heart attack thirty years earlier.

As we embarked on our project, Mike offered another insightful observation: "There is no such thing as writing, only re-writing." Totally on point.

Scott also pointed out that years earlier Mike served as his mentor, that he was bright, highly respected, and could not be outworked. That second opinion was most welcome, especially since it agreed with my original diagnosis.

We're both realistic. Our book might never get beyond "interesting little journal the two of them put together." But there will be others who will read it and come away enlightened with the knowledge that being a physician is not a job, it is a calling to heal and should never be wasted or taken for granted.

There will be patients who read it, become emboldened, and demand a role in their care. They will rightfully conclude that incessant questioning of their doctor is wholly acceptable. They have a right to a full discussion of the procedures and devices proposed to lengthen their years and increase the quality of their lives. They have a right to a frank assessment of risks associated with those procedures and devices. And they most assuredly have a right to insist on candor when the discussion turns to quality of life versus end of life. Timid patients who blindly relinquish control of their health because they are fearful of "offending the doctor" might also find some strength in these pages.

I frequently encounter the complaints of physicians who are retiring due to the mountains of required paperwork, government interference, and the necessity of converting to a system of electronic medical record keeping. My rejoinder to them is simple; the focus is between you and the patient—it always has been, and always will be. Nobody can interfere with that. If you became a physician for any other reason, then you have chosen the wrong career field. Hire someone to do the irritating work and concentrate on being a doctor.

I draw on the eloquence of Robert Frost to explain why the fighter still remains:

> "The woods are lovely, dark, and deep,
> but I have promises to keep,
> and miles to go before I sleep,
> and miles to go before I sleep."

Ike, Dick, and Mike

There are some interesting threads that weave their way through the three people we've enlisted to help tell our story; President Dwight D. Eisenhower, Vice President Dick Cheney, and the title deficient Mike Ranville.

All have a 'fish" connection. Eisenhower and Cheney were big fish in a big pond; and, while much of his labor was away from the public eye, Mike was an occasional big fish in a little pond.

All three could be described as "Type A" personalities. It is definite; we know the "Type A" behavior folks who have heart attacks enjoy a better survival rate. They are driven and the will to live is paramount to a successful recovery.

All three had a trusted family physician. Although Ike's physician completely missed the diagnosis, he didn't abandon his post at the bedside and enjoyed the confidence of the President.

All three had a Cardiologist who was trusted and the patients adhered to their Doctor's recommendations.

All three patients had a history of smoking: Ike, four packs a day, Dick Cheney, three packs a day, Mike a pack a day but much more when he was writing. It didn't take long for them to realize that survival was closely linked to removing tobacco from their life.

Ike probably never had his cholesterol checked but did change his diet, as did both Dick and Mike.

Exercise became part of their collective daily routine.

None of them shied from challenges and all three returned to their former high-stress jobs, refusing to seek or accept lightened workloads.

They thrived on the adrenaline that coursed through their daily schedules. It would have been more stressful for each of them to stay home and retrofit their lives to mundane tasks rather than to return to the familiarity of an environment they knew.

Most importantly, all three realized they were not immortal. The advice from people they came to know and trust was adhered to and instrumental in prompting dramatic changes in their lifestyles. Taken together, they present sterling evidence that medication can only do so much; if patients are willing to alter their lives for the better, fewer pharmaceuticals would be needed.

Ike was lucky and beat the bell curve at every point. He proved that genetics trump every other risk factor and if all of life is "genetics and environment" he fit the bill completely.

Dick and Mike benefitted tremendously from advances in knowledge and technology. All the tinker toys and tools of the interventionist and electrophysiologist, as well as lotions and potions, were assembled and used to the max. Both also fell outside the bell curve in that they beat the five-year survival for patients with a low ejection fraction. Dick received a LVAD. Then with one foot on a banana peel and the other in the grave he received a transplant, something that happens to less than 1 percent of patients that could benefit from this heroic and expensive operation. Mike's LVAD places him in an elite category; he is only one of one hundred and fifty patients in the state of Michigan and one of fifteen thousand worldwide to benefit from this very radical and expensive technology.

Personally I am lucky; I am blessed to have the genetic makeup that hopefully will never cause my cardiac bell to ring. Here at a small community hospital in Charlotte, Michigan, Mike was first admitted with his heart attack. He is alive today because a knowledgeable and caring family physician engineered a transfer to a larger, better equipped hospital. There he benefited from a facility that embraced and actively sought the latest technology. If it was available to Vice President Dick Cheney at the sophisticated environs of Georgetown University Hospital in Washington, D.C., then it was accessible to Mike Ranville at Ingham Medical. That alone speaks volumes to the availability of the most current advancements in cardiac care to all in need.

Rarely does a physician form the type of relationship I have with Mike. However, to a lesser degree, I strive to establish some type of personal relationship with every patient—and the patient's family.

Physicians have to deliver bad news; it comes with the territory. The virtue of the fact that patients are patients means they have some physical deficiency; that's why they came to us in the first place. I try to be tactful and not inflict unnecessary emotional harm, but steadfastly refuse to replace candor with saccharine when delivering news. No one benefits from the doctor who leaves the room with a patient under the false impression that all is well when it isn't. Granted, there are patients who can't or won't accept a straightforward assessment, but it should not be because the doctor was less than forthright.

Occasionally, though, we get to deliver good news.

One of my most satisfying moments occurs when a patient is sent to me with a new alleged cardiac diagnosis. After a thorough history and physical, and invoking a few of the tinker toys, I am able to tell them, "I don't know what my heart looks like, but I'll trade you now, because I know yours is stone cold normal." Or I'll say, "You don't need a cardiologist, go back to your family doctor because your heart is fine. " The smile on the patient's face, usually mirrored by an attending family member, is worth all the sixty-hour weeks and thousands of other patient encounters that do include structural heart disease.

But the real life practice of medicine in general, and cardiology in particular, is not like television where the weekly drama of life and death more often than not has a happy ending.

Occasionally, we see the tangible evidence of our efforts to add life to the years, not just years to the life, and the gratitude when we candidly acknowledge the difference. Yes, I keep the notes. Many are scribbled, barely legible, but that makes them all the more meaningful. It tells this ol' grinder that he brought some comfort to those in need. A sample is included below.

"Dr. James, to quote Eleanor Roosevelt—'yesterday is history, tomorrow is a mystery, and today is a gift.' Thank you for my continued good health."

"You were exactly right about Dad's philosophy of life. He didn't want to linger. He died peacefully."

"You were far more than a doctor to him, you were his friend."

"Thank you for coming to the funeral home. The family appreciated it so much, and I know he would have too."

"Thank you for everything. I ran five miles yesterday."

"Thank you for the quality of life you gave him. We have a picture of him riding a wave runner at age 88."

"The flowers were beautiful. Even more beautiful, though, was the fact that you sent them. You took care of _____ when he was alive, and now with the flowers you continue that care to his family. Thank you.

"_____ and the family always appreciated the candor about his condition."

While the doctor and the nurses are the most visible care givers to the patient, they are only the tip of the iceberg. There is a team of qualified and dedicated people functioning below that tip. Their commitment to excellence is no less valuable than that of the presiding physician.

When I was President of TCI, I was keenly aware of that iceberg. To reinforce the importance of teamwork, and to recognize the long hours that are an essential ingredient of the commitment to excellence, I came up with the idea to take all the employees and their families to Cedar Point for a day with TCI picking up the tab.

Including the families was fundamental to the invitation. Spouses and children had to know their Mom or Dad was an important person, vital to care we provided patients. Because they were important, they frequently had to work long hours. That message was delivered many times during the trip. Given the thank you letters, the TCI celebration at Cedar Point was noted and appreciated.

Another thank you surprise I initiated involved a dreary Friday. I reasoned it's tough to begin a weekend if for whatever reason Friday is particularly dismal. Occasionally, we would go to the bank, draw out the necessary amount to give each employee a $100 bill—"Just to say thank you for all your hard work."

Critical to both thank you gestures, and others, we meant it. They were not cosmetic pats on the back. Our success in caring for patients demanded excellence at all levels. We felt that excellence, no matter if it resided above or below the tip of the iceberg, should be rewarded.

The Next page...

Where do we go from here and what significance does all this have?

The thoughts above reflect my view of the world. That world, you may have already surmised, is governed by respect for human dignity. Further, Dr. Stein's sage counsel regarding "Life to Years versus Years to Life" is never far from my approach to end-of-life decisions.

I convene the discussion regarding end of life dynamics early in my relationship with heart failure patients. I bluntly – but hopefully with some modicum of tact – inform my patients they will enjoy a period of stability followed by a decline, sometimes rapid, where previously effective medication becomes ineffective.

There are alternatives; a continuous infusion of powerful drugs, a Left Ventricular Assist Device (LVAD), a transplant. But the overriding question becomes, "What expectations do you, the patient, have?"

Depending on the severity of your condition, do you want to do whatever is necessary to be with your family for one more Christmas? Or do you want to say, "Let nature take its course. I don't want my family's lasting memories of me to be as an infirmed onlooker, lacking the strength or ability to participate in the family festivities."

I also tell them that hospice has been a truly wonderful alternative. My gratitude abounds for the manner in which the nurses care for my patients and do so while preserving their dignity.

Our progress in caring for heart patients has been nothing short of astounding. We have seen more advancement in the past fifty years than in the previous five thousand years. We can stent arteries, even replace them. We can replace the heart's intricate electrical system and correct abnormal rhythms. We can replace valves. We can replace the entire heart with another. All of which would astound cardiologists and their patients of even a generation ago.

We are no longer preserving a community of television watchers. We are succeeding in the noble goal of adding "Life to Years."

Do not slide into the incoherence of end of life without having presented your wishes to your family or your physician. If you choose to have everything done, all the resources of medicine brought to bear, then say so. Those resources can add "years to your life."

But if you see little need for extending the inevitable and want to control your final days and ensure your dignity is preserved, then make those wishes known as well.

While your physician can provide a realistic assessment of your physical condition, your family can assume responsibility for your dignity.

The final chapter has yet to be written. I have every confidence that Mike's remaining years will be marked with accomplishment following his transplant.

Currently he is actively contributing to the cardiac community and rapidly becoming an articulate advocate for cardiac care in general.

He was invited by his LVAD surgeon, Dr. Jonathan Haft, to participate in a prestigious lecture given annually to medical students at the University of Michigan. Following Dr. Haft's remarks Mike answered questions regarding his decision to get the LVAD and the changes it brought about in his quality of life. By all accounts it was a lively and productive session.

He also spent an afternoon answering questions and acting as a "guinea pig patient" for a group of family practice residents. Some were blown away when they took a stethoscope to his chest and for the first time heard, not the rhythmic beat of a heart, but the humming of batteries propelling his LVAD.

On another occasion he was asked to hold forth on his LVAD experience to a Mid-west gathering of advanced heart failure physicians and nurses who were setting up clinics to care for patients in the LVAD pipeline.

And then most recently, Mike was asked to address the University of Michigan Cardiology community, both physicians and support staff. The audience was asked to fill out an evaluation form and, by all accounts, Mike's presentation was enthusiastically received.

Thank you, Mike Ranville, for being an Outlier and changing your lifestyle, taking your meds, and making me look good because of your success. All I did was my job, which is expected; you did the hard part.

Mike had a heart attack more than thirty years ago. He has been kept alive with new procedures, devices, and the latest in medicine. While Mike has done his part, I take great solace in knowing my efforts have brought "Life to his Years."

Not only has he been a prized patient, a successful example of what can be done to preserve life, he has also become a valued writing colleague and a good friend. I hope we can continue adding life to his years. And if all else fails, and our well of cardiac repairs run dry, I hope I have the courage to provide him and his family with the means to allow him a death with dignity.

The last chapter may yet be written.

CHAPTER TWENTY

THE FINAL PERSPECTIVE

Parting Message, Dr. Michael James:

Medical decisions are not easy. If they were, everyone from politicians to the 2:00 a.m. bar room philosopher would take credit for them. While not a politician—and no desire to become one—and my bar room philosophizing days long behind me, I offer my medical colleagues the following as a parting message:

1. Patients look to you for information and answers. Hesitation while filling that responsibility is not becoming. Therefore, trust yourself 100 percent of the time, your mom 50 percent of the time and no one else, ever.

2. When feeling sorry for yourself while rounding on a holiday or weekend, pause for just a moment to thank God you are on the right side of the white coat.

3. Don't make it more complicated than it already is. When assessing the health of a patient, they are either sick or not sick. If not sick, convince the patient. In many cases it is not the diagnosis the patient expects or wants. If sick, don't distort reality. Determine if, or how, you can make a difference.

4. Always remember, when you achieve a good result, the enemy of good is better.

5. To the patient, no procedure is routine. Before starting one, a little perspiration under the armpits and/or across the brow is a sign you are not approaching it as routine. That's good, both for you and the patient.

6. If a patient is truly asymptomatic it is difficult to make him more symptomatic by ordering unnecessary procedures. However there are certain conditions that asymptomatic patients have that do need immediate attention. So take this with a grain of salt.

7. Stay current. Medical journals may not move with the pace of a Grisham novel, but digesting them is critical to your role as an effective healer.

8. Errors of commission are forgivable. As a physician if you summoned all your knowledge and invested the appropriate time to make a decision, and it was wrong or harmed the patient, you are forgiven. But an error of omission—not investing the time or effort to analyze the medical situation, and the decision is wrong, that is wholly unacceptable.

9. Never turn an error of commission into an error of omission by covering up your mistake, admit it and move on.

10. Never – absolutely never – sacrifice candor for the fleeting smile of relief. It serves no one, least of all the patient and family.

From the Doctor for the patient:

1. If you are on more than four drugs, it's time to look for a new doctor.

2. If your doctor is offended by your decision to seek a second opinion, it's time to look for a new doctor.

3. If given a less than a sterling diagnosis, devote the next five minutes to feeling sorry for yourself. Then tell the doctor where to file that diagnosis, and then explain the filing directive: "For I have promises to keep, and miles to go before I sleep, and miles to go

before I sleep." Or feel free to quote me directly: "I still have a lot of tail to kick, and I intend to meet my quota.

4. Embrace the vision: "Every day a holiday, every meal a banquet."

I must ask for one more point of personal privilege. I present these thoughts not as an expression of ego, rather as a message to those who have graced my personal and professional life. I may never have another opportunity to tell you about the grinder who came to me early in life, remained ever at my side even when others had abandoned me, and would not accept failure or quitting as options. Someday you may have need of him.

When they tell you that you can't go to the high school of your choice, say just give me a shot, and then prove them wrong.

When you can't get into Notre Dame go to the University of Detroit and get a better education because you worked harder.

When they turn you down for Allopathic Medical School because you had a poor score on the Medical College Admission Test (MCAT), go to Osteopathic Medical School, do better, and return to teach and improve Osteopathic education.

When they won't let you become a cardiologist because you are an Osteopathic Physician, then do it, anyway possible.

When they tell you your patient is too old for a cardiac transplant then get it done somewhere, somehow, because you know it is the right thing to do.

From the patient to the world:

Heart disease is not the end of a productive life.

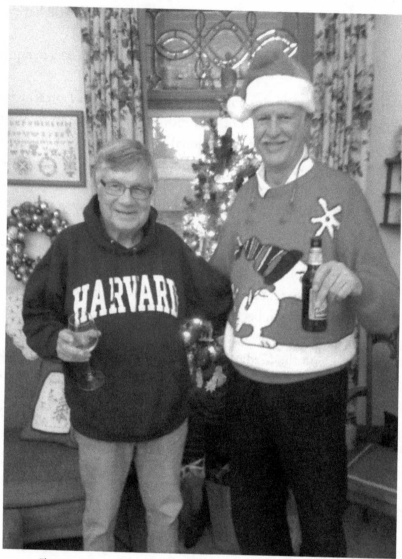

The two authors amidst the grueling task of preparing *Life to the Years*.

ACKNOWLEDGEMENTS

Dr. Michael J. James:

First and foremost I would like to acknowledge the contributions of my wife Wendy for the strong support she provided, from the book's inception to its completion. Far beyond just encouragement, her facility for detail and accuracy proved invaluable.

Thank you to my friend and colleague Dr. David Strobl. For years I watched him work miracles with heart patients and their diets, crucial to the productive life theme that courses through the book. Not only are his diets healthy, they are creative and doable. His chapter is a well-crafted message on the important role of diet, and a path to maintaining a healthy life style.

With some degree of personal pain, I recount in the book the passing of patient and close friend Ed Hardin, former President of Michigan State University. Pam Nyquist, President Hardin's daughter, eloquently captures the achievements that marked her father's remarkable life, and the dignity that characterized his death. Her comments added so much to our renderings on end-of-life decisions, a difficult chapter for both writing partner Mike Ranville and me.

Michael Ranville:

I would like to echo the sentiments of Dr. James and acknowledge Pam Nyquist. Long before Dr. James entered both our lives, I numbered Pam among my close friends in the Capitol—a sometimes brutal setting known more for its acquaintances not friends. My personal respect and admiration for her was enhanced by the account of her father's life and death.

It would be impossible to acknowledge the vast number of medical personnel who contributed to *keepin' me alive* to write this book. To name even a few, would be to neglect far too many who deserve mention. There is one notable exception, though…

Thank you, Dr. Michael James. Dr. Stein is surely smiling for you have carved a career that has added life to both our years.

And we both:

…acknowledge and deeply appreciate the skills of our editor Elisabeth Smith. She not only improved the book but her keen eye saved us from embarrassment a number of times.

…acknowledge the expertise of the entire Morgan James team. While our primary contacts were with David Hancock, Terry Whalin, Megan Malone and Niara Baskfield, we realize it was *a team of many* that guided the project from a scattered idea to that profound moment of actually holding a book in your hands. Writing a book is lot more than just writing a book.

…acknowledge both the scholarship and personal encouragement of Dr. Clarence G. Lasby. Clarence, your outstanding book, *Eisenhower's Heart Attack*, should be required reading for all Cardiac Fellows.

ABOUT THE AUTHORS

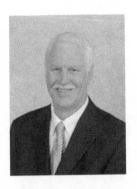

Michael James, D.O., FACC, is a Senior Partner at the Thoracic Cardiovascular Institute. He has served as a Clinical Professor on the faculty at Michigan State University since 1982. Dr. James is an avid skier and long-distance cyclist. He resides with his wife Wendy in Okemos, Michigan.

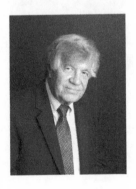

Michael Ranville worked in the political arena for more than 35 years, primarily as a researcher, speechwriter and lobbyist. He retired in 2005 to pursue a career in writing. He publishes articles and writes speeches for political candidates, educators and the business community. He is nearing completion of a new book, *Another Page in History*.

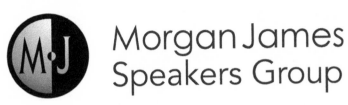

Morgan James
Speakers Group

We connect Morgan James published
authors with live and online events
and audiences who will benefit
from their expertise.

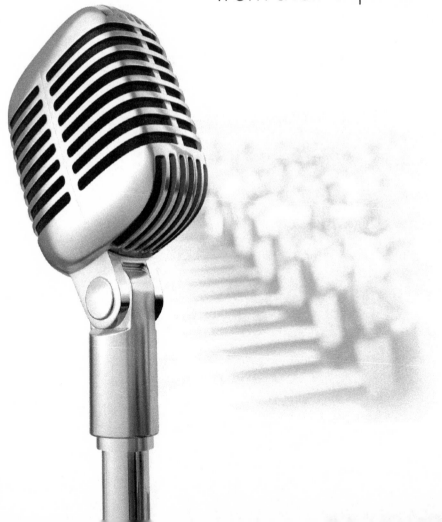

 Morgan James makes all of our titles available
through the Library for All Charity Organization.

www.LibraryForAll.org

CPSIA information can be obtained
at www.ICGtesting.com
Printed in the USA
BVHW08s0123140618
519030BV00001B/8/P